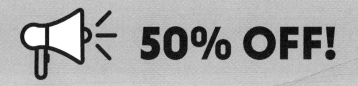 **50% OFF!**

MW01077551

ATI TEAS 7® ONLINE TEST PREP COURSE

We consider it an honor and a privilege that you chose our ATI TEAS 7® Study Guide. As a way of showing our appreciation and to help us better serve you, we have partnered with Mometrix Test Preparation to offer you 50% off their online ATI TEAS 7® Prep Course.

Mometrix has structured their online course to perfectly complement your printed study guide. Many ATI TEAS 7® courses are needlessly expensive and don't deliver enough value. With their course, you get access to the best ParaPro prep material, and you only pay half price.

WHAT'S IN THE ATI TEAS 7® TEST PREP COURSE?

- ✓ **ATI TEAS 7® Study Guide**: Get access to content that complements your study guide.

- ✓ **Progress Tracker**: Their customized course allows you to check off content you have studied or feel confident with.

- ✓ **2650+ Practice Questions**: With 2650+ practice questions and lesson reviews, you can test yourself again and again to build confidence.

- ✓ **ATI TEAS 7® Flashcards**: Their course includes a flashcard mode consisting of over 310 content cards to help you study.

TO RECEIVE THIS DISCOUNT, VISIT THE WEBSITE AT

link.mometrix.com/teas

USE THE DISCOUNT CODE:
STARTSTUDYING

SCAN HERE

IF YOU HAVE ANY QUESTIONS OR CONCERNS, PLEASE
CONTACT MOMETRIX AT SUPPORT@MOMETRIX.COM

Mometrix
ONLINE COURSES

FREE VIDEO

Essential Test Tips Video from Trivium Test Prep!

Thank you for purchasing from Trivium Test Prep!
We're honored to help you prepare for your exam.
To show our appreciation, we're offering a

FREE *Essential Test Tips* Video

Our video includes 35 test preparation strategies that will make you successful
on your big exam. All we ask is that you email us your feedback and describe
your experience with our product. Amazing, awful, or just so-so:
we want to hear what you have to say!

> To receive your **FREE *Essential Test Tips* Video**, please email us at
> **5star@triviumtestprep.com.**

Include "Free 5 Star" in the subject line and the following information in your email:

1. The title of the product you purchased.
2. Your rating from 1 – 5 (with 5 being the best).
3. Your feedback about the product, including how our materials helped you meet
   your goals and ways in which we can improve our products.
4. Your full name and shipping address so we can send your
   FREE *Essential Test Tips* Video.

If you have any questions or concerns please feel free to contact us directly at:
5star@triviumtestprep.com.

Thank you!
– Trivium Test Prep Team

ATI TEAS® 7th Edition 2025-2026 Study Guide:

1200+ Practice Test Questions and TEAS Exam Prep

B. Hettinger

Table of Contents

Online Resources vii

Introduction ix

What's on the ATI TEAS? ix
How Do I Register for the TEAS? x
How Is the TEAS Scored? x
When Will I Receive My TEAS Score? x
What's a Good Score on the TEAS? xi
How to Use This Guide..........................xi
About Trivium Test Prep xi

Part 1 Reading 1

1 Reading Text 3

Key Ideas and Details 3
Craft and Structure.............................10
Integration of Knowledge and Ideas..............13
Vocabulary....................................18
Answer Key 24

2 Reading Graphics 27

Graphs..27
Maps..29
Scale Readings 30
Product Information............................32
Using Graphics 33
Answer Key 35

Part 2 Mathematics 37

3 Numbers and Operations 39

Arithmetic Operations 39

Exponents and Radicals 40
Order of Operations 42
Fractions 43
Decimals 44
Comparison of Rational Numbers...............45
Ratios and Proportions 46
Percents 47
Estimation and Rounding 48
Answer Key 50

4 Algebra 53

Expressions and Equations.....................53
Equations.....................................54
Graphing Linear Equations on a
Coordinate Plane..............................55
Inequalities 57
Building Equations............................58
Absolute Value 59
Answer Key 61

5 Geometry 63

Units of Measurement 63
Lines and Angles 65
Two-Dimensional Shapes 66
Three-Dimensional Shapes.....................69
Congruency and Similarity 71
Answer Key 72

6 Statistics 75

Measures of Central Tendency.................75
Measures of Dispersion........................76
Data Presentation.............................77
Data Distribution.............................81

Answer Key 83

Part 3 Science 85

7 Human Anatomy and Physiology 87

The Biological Hierarchy 87
Directional Terminology 88
Body Cavities and Planes 89
The Cardiovascular System 91
The Respiratory System 94
The Nervous System 97
The Skeletal System 100
The Muscular System 103
The Immune System 106
The Digestive System 108
The Urinary System 111
The Reproductive System 112
The Endocrine System 115
The Integumentary System 118
Homeostasis 120
Answer Key 122

8 Biology 125

Biological Macromolecules 125
Nucleic Acids 129
Genetics 134
The Cell 140
Mitosis and Meiosis 143
Microorganisms and Infectious Disease 146
Answer Key 148

9 Chemistry 151

The Structure of the Atom 151
Electron Configuration 152
The Periodic Table of the Elements 154
Chemical Bonding 158
Physical and Chemical Properties 160
States of Matter 161
Properties of Water 163

Acids and Bases 164
Solutions 166
Chemical Reactions 168
Answer Key 177

10 Scientific Reasoning 179

Systems 179
Scientific Investigations 180
Laws and Theories 181
Sources of Error 181
The Scientific Method 181
Answer Key 183

Part 4 English and Language Usage 185

11 Parts of Speech 187

Nouns and Pronouns 187
Verbs 188
Adjectives and Adverbs 191
Other Parts of Speech 192
Answer Key 194

12 Sentence Structure 195

Phrases 195
Clauses 196
Punctuation 197
Capitalization 199
Homophones and Spelling 200
Answer Key 205

13 Writing 207

The Writing Process 207
Organizing Writing 209
Revising Informal and Formal Language 209
Avoiding Bias 210
Answer Key 212

14 Practice Test 213

Answer Key 237

Online Resources

Trivium Test Prep includes online resources with the purchase of this study guide to help you fully prepare for your ATI TEAS, Version 7 exam.

Practice Test

In addition to the practice test included in this book, we also offer an online exam. Since many exams today are computer based, practicing your test-taking skills on the computer is a great way to prepare.

Review Questions

Need more practice? Our review questions use a variety of formats to help you memorize key terms and concepts.

Flash Cards

Trivium Test Prep's flash cards allow you to review important terms easily on your computer or smartphone.

Cheat Sheets

Review the core skills you need to master the exam with easy-to-read Cheat Sheets.

From Stress to Success

Watch "From Stress to Success," a brief but insightful YouTube video that offers the tips, tricks, and secrets experts use to score higher on the exam.

Feedback

Let us know what you think!

Access these materials at:

www.triviumtestprep.com/ati-teas-online-resources

Introduction

Congratulations on your decision to join the field of nursing—few other professions are so rewarding! By purchasing this book, you've already taken the first step toward succeeding in your career. The next step is to do well on the Assessment Technologies Institute (ATI) Test of Essential Academic Skills (TEAS), which will require you to demonstrate knowledge of high school-level reading, writing, math, and science.

This book will walk you through the important concepts in each of these subjects and provide you with inside information on test strategies and tactics. Even if it's been years since you graduated from high school or cracked open a textbook, don't worry; this book contains everything you'll need for the ATI TEAS.

What's on the ATI TEAS?

For the ATI TEAS, you will have **3 hours and 30 minutes** to answer **170 questions. The questions will be divided into four sections:**

- Reading (39 questions)
- Math (34 questions)
- Science (44 questions)
- English and Language Usage (33 questions)

Each section includes pretest questions that are unscored. These 20 questions are included by the test makers to gauge their appropriateness for the exam. Pretest questions do not count toward your score; however, you won't know which questions are unscored, so you need to answer all of them.

WHAT'S on the TEAS?

CONTENT AREA	SUB-CONTENT AREAS	NUMBER OF QUESTIONS
Reading	Key ideas and details	15
	Craft and structure	9
	Integration of knowledge and ideas	15
Math	Numbers and algebra	18
	Measurement and data	16
Science	Human anatomy and physiology	18
	Biology	9
	Chemistry	8
	Scientific reasoning	9
English and Language Usage	Conventions of standard English	12
	Knowledge of language	11
	Using language and vocabulary to express ideas in writing	10
Pretest Questions		20
Total		170 questions

How Do I Register for the TEAS?

The TEAS is administered by ATI, and you can register for the test on their website (www.atitesting.com). You can choose to take the test online, at a university campus, or at a PSI national testing center. Before you register, check with the institutions where you plan to apply—they may ask for scores from certain locations.

How Is the TEAS Scored?

On your TEAS score report, you will see your percentile rank for each of the content and sub-content areas. A percentile rank tells you how you performed compared to other test takers. For example, if you score in the seventy-eighth percentile, that means you did better than 78 percent of all test takers.

When Will I Receive My TEAS Score?

The time frame in which you receive your score depends on where you take the test. If you take it online or on a campus, you will likely be able to see your score immediately; however, if you test at a PSI center or complete a paper-and-pencil version of the test, you will see your results in your ATI account within 24 to 72 hours.

What's a Good Score on the TEAS?

There's no "good" or "bad" score on the TEAS. Schools consider TEAS scores as part of a comprehensive application process. Each school has its own requirements for TEAS scores, so check with the schools where you plan to apply.

How to Use This Guide

This guide is not meant to waste your time on superfluous information or concepts you've already learned. Instead, we hope you will use this guide to develop critical test-taking skills and focus on the concepts YOU need to master for the test. To support this effort, the guide provides:

- organized concepts with detailed explanations
- practice questions with worked-through solutions
- key test-taking strategies
- a simulated one-on-one tutor experience
- tips, tricks, and test secrets

Because we have eliminated filler and fluff, you'll be able to work through the guide at a significantly faster pace than you would with other test prep books. By allowing you to focus only on those concepts that will increase your score, this guide makes your study time shorter and more effective.

The chapters in this book are divided into a review of the topics covered on the exam. This is not intended to teach you everything you'll see on the test—there is no way to cram all of that material into one book! Instead, we are going to help you recall information that you've already learned and, more importantly, we'll show you how to apply that knowledge. With time, practice, and determination, you'll be well prepared for test day.

About Trivium Test Prep

Trivium Test Prep uses industry professionals with decades' worth of knowledge in their fields, proven with degrees and honors in law, medicine, business, education, the military, and more, to produce high quality test prep books for students.

Our study guides are specifically designed to increase any student's score. Our books are also shorter and more concise than typical study guides, so you can increase your score while significantly decreasing your study time.

Reading

The ATI TEAS Reading section will require you to answer questions about text passages and graphics such as maps, drawings, or charts. These questions will fall into three categories:

- **Key ideas and details** questions ask about the main idea of the passage and the details that support that main idea.

- **Craft and structure** questions ask about the craft of writing, including organization of the text, word choice, and the author's purpose.

- **Integration of knowledge and ideas** questions require drawing conclusions from passages and integrating information from multiple sources.

1 | Reading Text

The majority of the questions on the TEAS Reading section will refer to **passages**, which are short texts about a nonfiction topic. You will be asked to read the passage and then answer questions about the passage's content, how it is constructed, and what conclusions you can draw from it. You will also see standalone questions in the Reading section that test your understanding of research skills and writing mechanics.

Key Ideas and Details

The Main Idea

The **main idea** of a text is the argument that the author is trying to make about a particular **topic**. Every sentence in a passage should support or address the main idea in some way.

Consider a political election. A candidate is running for office and plans to deliver a speech asserting her position on tax reform, which is that taxes should be lowered. The topic of the speech is tax reform, and the main idea is that taxes should be lowered. The candidate is going to assert this in her speech, and support it with examples proving why lowering taxes would benefit the public and how it could be accomplished.

Other candidates may have different perspectives on the same topic. They may believe that higher taxes are necessary or that current taxes are adequate. Their speeches, while on the same topic of tax reform, would probably have different main ideas supported by different examples and evidence.

Let's look at an example passage to see how to identify the topic and main idea.

Babe Didrikson Zaharias, one of the most decorated female athletes of the twentieth century, is an inspiration for everyone. Born in 1911 in Port Arthur, Texas, Zaharias lived in a time when women were considered second class to men, but she never let that stop her from becoming a champion. Babe was one of seven children in a poor

 HELPFUL HINT

Topic: The subject of the passage. **Main idea:** The argument the writer is making about the topic.

immigrant family and was competitive from an early age. As a child she excelled at most things she tried, particularly sports. In fact, she left high school early in order to play amateur basketball. She played basketball for two years, and soon after began training in track and field. Despite being a relative newcomer, Zaharias represented the United States in the 1932 Los Angeles Olympics. At the games, she won two gold medals and one silver for track and field events.

The topic of this paragraph is obviously Babe Zaharias—the whole passage describes events from her life. Determining the main idea, however, requires a little more analysis. To figure out the main idea, consider what the writer is saying about Zaharias. The passage describes her life, but the main idea of the paragraph is what it says about her accomplishments. The writer is saying that Zaharias is someone to admire. That is the main idea and what unites all the information in the paragraph.

PRACTICE QUESTIONS

Tourists flock to Yellowstone National Park each year to view the geysers that bubble and erupt throughout it. What most of these tourists do not know is that these geysers are formed by a caldera, a hot crater in the earth's crust that was created by a series of three eruptions from an ancient supervolcano. These eruptions, which began 2.1 million years ago, spewed between 1,000 and 2,450 cubic kilometers of volcanic matter at such a rate that the volcano's magma chamber collapsed, creating the craters.

1. Which of the following is the topic of the passage?
   A) tourists
   B) geysers
   C) volcanic eruptions
   D) supervolcanoes

The Battle of the Little Bighorn (1876), commonly called Custer's Last Stand, was a battle between the Lakota, the Northern Cheyenne, the Arapaho, and the Seventh Cavalry Regiment of the US Army. Led by war leaders Crazy Horse and Chief Gall and the religious leader Sitting Bull, the allied tribes of the Plains Indians decisively defeated their US foes. Two hundred sixty-eight US soldiers were killed, including General George Armstrong Custer, two of his brothers, his nephew, his brother-in-law, and six Indian scouts.

2. Which of the following is the main idea of the passage?
   A) Most of General Custer's family died in the Battle of the Little Bighorn.
   B) During the nineteenth century, the US Army often fought with Indian tribes.
   C) Sitting Bull and George Custer were fierce enemies.
   D) The Battle of the Little Bighorn was a significant victory for the Plains Indians.

Topic and Summary Sentences

The topic, and sometimes the main idea of a paragraph, is introduced in the **topic sentence**. The topic sentence usually appears early in a passage. The first sentence in the example paragraph about Babe Zaharias states the topic and main idea: "Babe Didrikson Zaharias, one of the most decorated female athletes of the twentieth century, is an inspiration for everyone."

Even though paragraphs generally begin with a topic sentence, writers sometimes build up to the topic sentence by using supporting details to generate interest or to build an argument. Be alert for paragraphs that do not include a clear topic sentence.

There may also be a **summary sentence** at the end of a passage. As its name suggests, this type of sentence sums up the passage, often by restating the main idea and the author's key evidence supporting it.

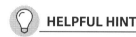

HELPFUL HINT

On the TEAS, you may be asked to summarize a passage. An effective **summary** of a passage will restate the main idea and the most important supporting details.

PRACTICE QUESTION

> The Constitution of the United States establishes a series of limits to rein in centralized power. "Separation of powers" distributes federal authority among three branches: the executive, the legislative, and the judicial. The system of "checks and balances" prevents any one branch from usurping power. "States' rights" are protected under the Constitution from too much encroachment by the federal government. "Enumeration of powers" names the specific and few powers the federal government has. These four restrictions have helped sustain the American republic for over two centuries.

3. Which of the following is the passage's topic sentence?
   A) "These four restrictions have helped sustain the American republic for over two centuries."
   B) "The Constitution of the United States establishes a series of limits to rein in centralized power."
   C) "'Enumeration of powers' names the specific and few powers the federal government has."
   D) "The system of 'checks and balances' prevents any one branch from usurping power."

Supporting Details

Supporting details reinforce the author's main idea. Let's look again at the passage about athlete Babe Zaharias.

> Babe Didrikson Zaharias, one of the most decorated female athletes of the twentieth century, is an inspiration for everyone. Born in 1911 in Port Arthur, Texas, Zaharias lived in a time when women were considered second class to men, but she never let that stop her from becoming a champion. Babe was one of seven children in a poor immigrant family and was competitive from an early age. As a child she excelled at most things she tried, particularly sports. In fact, she left high school early in order to play amateur basketball. She played

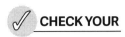

CHECK YOUR UNDERSTANDING

Which signal words can you find in this passage? What function are they performing (e.g., introducing information, showing sequence)?

basketball for two years, and soon after began training in track and field. Despite being a relative newcomer, Zaharias represented the United States in the 1932 Los Angeles Olympics. At the games, she won two gold medals and one silver for track and field events.

The main idea of the passage is that Zaharias is someone to admire. This idea is introduced in the opening sentence. The rest of the paragraph provides details that support this idea. These details include the circumstances of her childhood, her early success at sports, and the medals she won at the Olympics.

When looking for supporting details, be alert for **signal words**. These words or phrases tell you that a supporting fact or idea will follow and so can be helpful in identifying supporting details. Signal words can also help you rule out certain sentences as the main idea or topic sentence: if a sentence begins with one of these phrases, it will likely be too specific to be a main idea. Some common signal words are listed below.

- adding information: also, furthermore, in addition, too
- comparing: like, likewise, similarly
- contrasting: alternatively, instead of, on the other hand, unlike
- give an example: for example, for instance, in other words, in particular
- sequence: after, before, first/second, next, then
- show cause and effect: because, so, therefore, consequently

When analyzing supporting details, it's important to differentiate between a fact and an opinion. A **fact** is a statement or thought that can be proven to be true. The statement "Wednesday comes after Tuesday" is a fact—you can point to a calendar to prove it. In contrast, an **opinion** is an assumption, not based in fact, that cannot be proven to be true. The assertion that "television is more entertaining than feature films" is an opinion—people will disagree on this, and there is no reference you can use to prove or disprove it.

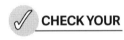

CHECK YOUR UNDERSTANDING

Which of the following phrases are associated with opinions? *for example, studies have shown, I believe, in fact, it's possible that*

PRACTICE QUESTIONS

From so far away, it's easy to imagine the surface of our solar system's planets as enigmas—how could we ever know what those far-flung planets really look like? It turns out, however, that scientists have a number of tools at their disposal that allow them to paint detailed pictures of many planets' surfaces. The topography of Venus, for example, has been explored by several space probes, including the Russian Venera landers and NASA's *Magellan* orbiter. In addition to these long-range probes, NASA has also used its series of orbiting telescopes to study distant planets. These four massively powerful telescopes include the famous Hubble Space Telescope as well as the Compton Gamma Ray Observatory, the Chandra X-Ray Observatory, and the Spitzer Space Telescope. Such powerful telescopes aren't just found in space: NASA makes use of Earth-based telescopes as well. Scientists at the National Radio Astronomy Observatory in Charlottesville, Virginia, have spent decades using radio imaging to build an incredibly detailed portrait of Venus's surface.

4. According to the passage, which of the following is a space probe used to explore the surface of Venus?

    A) *Magellan* orbiter

    B) Hubble Space Telescope

    C) Spitzer Space Telescope

    D) National Radio Astronomy Observatory

5. If true, which detail could be added to the previous passage to support the author's assertion that scientists use many different technologies to study the surface of planets?

    A) Because Earth's atmosphere blocks X-rays, gamma rays, and infrared radiation, NASA needed to put telescopes in orbit above the atmosphere.

    B) In 2015, NASA released a map of Venus that was created by compiling images from orbiting telescopes and long-range space probes.

    C) NASA is currently using the *Curiosity* and *Opportunity* rovers to look for signs of ancient life on Mars.

    D) NASA has spent over $2.5 billion to build, launch, and repair the Hubble Space Telescope.

Directions and Events in a Sequence

Some questions on the TEAS will require you to follow a set of simple directions. These directions can be given in either paragraph or list format. Each step, or direction, usually includes specific instructions that must be remembered in order to complete the subsequent steps. The directions will require you to manipulate quantities (such as money or numbers of items) or shapes to reach the final answer.

Sequence words explain how events fall in chronological or logical order. For example, the transition *subsequently* tells you that one event happened *after* another. The phrase *at the same time* shows that two events happened concurrently. On the TEAS, you will need to pay attention to sequence words in order to follow directions or determine in what order events in a passage occurred.

Sequence words in a sentence or paragraph act as guideposts to the action. Common sequence words to look out for include:

- after
- at the same time
- before
- concurrently
- currently
- first
- later
- next
- recently
- second

 HELPFUL HINT

Write out the new answer for each step as you finish it so you can easily check your work.

- since
- subsequently
- then
- while

PRACTICE QUESTIONS

6. Read the paragraph, then answer the question.

[1] First, mobile dining took a new form in the 1900s, as the invention of motorized transportation began to transform the industry. [2] Ice cream trucks then followed in the 1950s, serving children and adults alike cold treats on hot summer afternoons. [3] Finally, in the 1960s, large food service trucks called "roach coaches" began to pop up near densely populated urban areas, often serving cheap meals from grungy kitchens.

Upon reviewing the previous paragraph and realizing that some information had been left out, the writer composes the following sentence:

During the 1940s and WWII, mobile canteens popped up near Army bases to serve quick, easy meals to the troops.

Where would the most logical placement for this sentence be?

A) before sentence one

B) before sentence two

C) before sentence three

D) after sentence three

7. Starting with three red apples and one green apple in a basket, how many apples are in the basket after following the directions below?
1. Remove one red apple.
2. Add one green apple.
3. Add one red apple.
4. Add one green apple.
5. Remove two red apples.
6. Remove one green apple.
7. Add three red apples.
8. Add two green apples.

A) four red apples and two green apples

B) four red apples and four green apples

C) two red apples and three green apples

D) zero red apples and three green apples

8. There are twelve gallons of fuel in a tank. After following the directions below, how many gallons of fuel are left in the tank?
1. Use one gallon to drive to work.
2. Use one gallon to drive home.
3. Use half a gallon to drive the kids to soccer practice.
4. Use half a gallon to drive to the grocery store.
5. Use two gallons to drive back home.

A) two gallons

B) five and a half gallons

C) seven gallons

D) eight and a half gallons

Indexes and Tables of Contents

An **index** is an alphabetical list of topics, and their associated page numbers, covered in a text. A **table of contents** is an outline of a text that includes topics, organized by page number. Both of these can be used to look up information, but they have slightly different purposes. An index helps readers determine where in the text they can find specific details. A table of contents shows the general arrangement of the text.

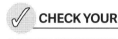 **CHECK YOUR**

UNDERSTANDING

When navigating a book, when would it be better to use an index instead of the table of contents?

PRACTICE QUESTIONS

9. The index below is taken from a nursing textbook.

> Nursing, pp. 189 – 296
>
> certification, pp. 192 – 236
>
> code of ethics, pp. 237 – 291
>
> procedures, pp. 292 – 296

According to the index, where will the reader find information about the nursing code of ethics?

A) pp. 237 – 291

B) pp. 189 – 296

C) pp. 292 – 296

D) pp. 189 – 236

10. The table of contents below is taken from a math textbook.

Table of Contents	
Chapter 1: Pre-Algebra	5
Chapter 2: Algebra	35
Chapter 3: Geometry	115
Chapter 4: Calculus	175

A student has been assigned a set of homework questions from page 125. What topic will the questions cover?

A) pre-algebra

B) algebra

C) geometry

D) calculus

Text Features

Text features are stylistic elements used to clarify, add meaning, or differentiate. Examples of text features include bold, italicized, or underlined fonts, and bulleted or numbered lists.

Bold fonts are generally used for emphasis. Italics should be used for titles of long works, such as novels, movies, books, magazines, and plays. They are also used to denote a foreign word or phrase. Note that italicized fonts and underlined fonts serve similar purposes and are often used interchangeably. Underlining is more commonly used in handwritten documents.

PRACTICE QUESTION

11. Which of the following sentences properly uses italics?
    A) We enjoyed our vacation in *Sacramento, California.*
    B) Adam ate two plates of *pasta with meatballs.*
    C) Angela's favorite book is *The Art of War.*
    D) The traffic on *Main Street* is terrible during rush hour.

Craft and Structure

Types of Passages

Authors typically write with a purpose. Sometimes referred to as "authorial intention," an author's purpose lets the reader know why the author is writing and what he or she would like to accomplish. There are many reasons an author might write, but most write for one of four reasons:

- to **entertain** the reader or tell a story
- to **persuade** the reader of their opinion
- to **describe** something, such as a person, place, thing, or event
- to **explain** a process or procedure

Identifying an author's purpose can be tricky, but the writing itself often gives clues. For example, if an author's purpose is to entertain, the writing may include vivid characters; exciting plot twists; or beautiful, figurative language. On the other hand, if an author wishes to persuade the reader, the passage may present an argument or contain convincing examples that support the author's point of view. An author who wishes to describe a person, place, or event may include lots of details as well as plenty of adjectives and adverbs. Finally, the author whose purpose is to explain a process or procedure may include step-by-step instructions or might present information in a sequence.

Related to authorial intention are the different **modes** of written materials. A short story, for example, is meant to entertain, while an online news article is designed to inform the public about a current event.

Each of these different types of writing has a specific name. On the ATI TEAS, you will be asked to identify which of these categories a passage fits into:

- **Narrative writing** tells a story (novel, short story, play).
- **Informational** (or **expository**) **writing** informs people (newspaper and magazine articles).
- **Technical writing** explains something (product manual, instructions).
- **Persuasive writing** tries to convince the reader of something (opinion column or a blog).

PRACTICE QUESTIONS

One of my summer reading books was *Mockingjay*. I was captivated by the adventures of the main character and the complicated plot of the book. However, I would argue that the ending didn't reflect the excitement of the story. Given what a powerful personality the main character has, I felt like the ending didn't do her justice.

12. Which of the following BEST captures the author's purpose?

A) to explain the plot of the novel *Mockingjay*

B) to persuade the reader that the ending of *Mockingjay* is weak

C) to list the novels she read during the summer

D) to explain why the ending of a novel is important

Elizabeth closed her eyes and braced herself on the armrests that divided her from her fellow passengers. Takeoff was always the worst part for her. The revving of the engines, the way her stomach dropped as the plane lurched upward: It made her feel sick. Then, she had to watch the world fade away beneath her, getting smaller and smaller until it was just her and the clouds hurtling through the sky. Sometimes (but only sometimes) it just had to be endured. She focused on the thought of her sister's smiling face and her new baby nephew as the plane slowly pulled onto the runway.

13. Which of the following BEST describes the mode of the passage?

A) narrative

B) expository

C) technical

D) persuasive

Text Structure

Authors can structure passages in a number of different ways. These distinct organizational patterns, referred to as **text structure**, use the logical relationships between ideas to improve the readability and coherence of a text. The most common ways passages are organized include:

- **problem-solution**: The author outlines a problem and then discusses a solution.
- **comparison-contrast**: The author presents two situations and then discusses the similarities and differences.

- **cause-effect**: The author recounts an action and then discusses the resulting effects.
- **descriptive**: The author describes an idea, object, person, or other item in detail.

PRACTICE QUESTION

> The issue of public transportation has begun to haunt the fast-growing cities of the southern United States. Unlike their northern counterparts, cities like Atlanta, Dallas, and Houston have long promoted growth out and not up—these are cities full of sprawling suburbs and single-family homes, not densely concentrated skyscrapers and apartment buildings. What to do then, when all those suburbanites need to get into the central business districts for work? For a long time, it seemed highways were the answer: twenty-lane-wide expanses of concrete that would allow commuters to move from home to work and back again. But these modern miracles have become time-sucking, pollution-spewing nightmares. The residents of these cities may not like it, but it's time for them to turn toward public transport like trains and buses if they want their cities to remain livable.

14. The organization of this passage can BEST be described as

A) a comparison of two similar ideas.

B) a description of a place.

C) a discussion of several effects all related to the same cause.

D) a discussion of a problem followed by a suggested solution.

Point of View

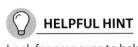 **HELPFUL HINT**

Look for pronouns to help identify which point of view a sentence is using.

Point of view is the perspective from which the action in a story is told. By carefully selecting a particular point of view, writers can control what their readers know. Most literature is written in either the **first person** or **third person** point of view. Some writing uses the second person point of view.

With the **first person point of view**, the action is narrated by a character within the story, which can make it feel more believable and authentic to the reader. However, the reader's knowledge and understanding are constrained by what the narrator notices and influenced by what the narrator thinks and values.

A **third person point of view** uses a narrative voice outside the action of the story. A third person narrator might be fully omniscient (able to see into the minds of the characters and share what they are thinking and feeling), partially omniscient (able to see into the minds of just one or a few characters), or limited (unable to see into the minds of any of the characters and only able to share what can be seen and heard).

The first person point of view is best used when the writer's personal experiences, feelings, and opinions are an important element. Second person point of view is best for types of writing in which the author directly addresses the reader. Third person point of view is most common in formal and academic writing; it creates distance between the writer and the reader. A sentence's point of view has to remain consistent throughout the sentence.

TABLE 1.1. Point of View

PERSON	PRONOUNS USED	WHO'S ACTING?	EXAMPLE
First	I, we	the writer	I take my time when shopping for shoes.
Second	you	the reader	You prefer to shop online.
Third	he, she, it, they	the subject	She buys shoes from her cousin's store.

PRACTICE QUESTION

15. Read the paragraph, then answer the question that follows.

> Empathy is different from mimicry or sympathy—it is neither imitating someone else's emotions nor feeling concern for their suffering. Empathy is much more complex; it is the ability to actually share and comprehend the emotions of others.

From which perspective is this text written?

A) first person

B) second person

C) third person

D) There is not enough information to determine the perspective.

Integration of Knowledge and Ideas

Drawing Conclusions and Making Inferences

To draw a **conclusion**, the reader must identify a statement that logically follows the ideas presented in a piece of writing. An **inference** is a little bit different: it is an educated guess readers make based on the writing *and* their own knowledge. Let's look at an example.

> Addressing climate change is essential if we want to leave our children a habitable world. This issue cannot be resolved without addressing the underlying cause of climate change—our reliance on fossil fuels, including oil, coal, and natural gas. Together, these sources account for 80 percent of US energy consumption.

A logical conclusion to draw from this passage is that the author supports policies that decrease the use of fossil fuels. The author states that fossil fuels are the "underlying cause" of climate change that must be addressed.

Readers can also make inferences by drawing on their own knowledge. For example, the reader might infer that the author supports wind energy as an alternative to fossil fuels. Note that the passage does not explicitly mention wind energy—readers must use their own knowledge to infer this information.

On the TEAS, questions may explicitly ask you to draw a conclusion or make an inference. They may also ask you to make inferences indirectly with questions about the author's intention or beliefs. On a nonfiction passage, for example, you might be asked which statement the author would agree with.

PRACTICE QUESTION

> Exercise is critical for healthy development in children. Today in the United States, there is an epidemic of poor childhood health; many of these children will face further illnesses in adulthood that are due to poor diet and lack of exercise now. This is a problem for all Americans, especially with the rising cost of health care.
>
> It is vital that school systems and parents encourage children to engage in a minimum of thirty minutes of cardiovascular exercise each day, mildly increasing their heart rate for a sustained period. This is proven to decrease the likelihood of developmental diabetes, obesity, and a multitude of other health problems. Also, children need a proper diet, rich in fruits and vegetables, so they can develop physically and learn healthy eating habits early on.

16. Which of the following statements might the author of this passage agree with?

A) Adults who do not have healthy eating habits should be forced to pay more for health care.

B) Schools should be required by federal law to provide vegetables with every meal.

C) Healthy eating habits can only be learned at home.

D) Schools should encourage students to bring lunches from home.

 DID YOU KNOW?

Primary sources are usually written by people who have directly experienced an event. Secondary sources are written by people who did NOT experience the event themselves.

Citing Sources

The ATI TEAS Reading section also includes questions about using sources for research. You will need to be able to differentiate between primary and secondary sources, and identify a useful and credible source of information.

The terms *primary source* and *secondary source* describe an author's relationship to their topic. A **primary source** is an unaltered piece of writing that was composed during the time the events being described took place; these texts are often written by the people involved in those events. A **secondary source** might address the same topic but provides extra commentary or analysis. These texts can be written by people not directly involved in the events. For example, a book written by a political candidate to inform people about their stand on an issue is a primary source; an online article written by a journalist analyzing how that position will affect the election is a secondary source.

When researching a topic, it is necessary to determine whether or not any given source is credible. A source is credible if it is from an expert authority and is free from bias. Credible sources provide research that is trustworthy because the information has been fact-checked. Such sources include peer-reviewed journals (journals that ask other experts to review content before it is published) and websites from reputable institutions such as the World Health Organization or the American Academy of Pediatrics. Less credible sources include personal blogs, opinion pieces, and online message boards.

How can you tell if a source is credible? Ask yourself the following questions:

- Is the article from a peer-reviewed journal? (Most research journals will identify themselves as peer-reviewed on their website or in the journal itself. You may also limit your library database searches to include only peer-reviewed research.)

- Is the article recent? (Articles that are over a decade old may contain information that is out of date or that has been proven inaccurate.)

- Is the author trustworthy? (Is the author of the article listed? Does the author have academic credentials, such as a PhD, or hold an academic post? Is the author free from bias or does the author seem to promote a particular political view or personal agenda?)

PRACTICE QUESTIONS

17. The students in Professor Johnson's class are searching for secondary sources for a paper on the polio vaccine. Which of the following might they consult?

A) an interview with a person who has been diagnosed with polio

B) pictures of patients who have received the polio vaccine

C) a journal article on the rate of polio inoculation in the United States

D) an interview with a doctor who specializes in the treatment of polio

18. Cynthia wants to research the effectiveness of soap from different manufacturers. Where should she look for this information?

A) a blog

B) the manufacturer's website

C) an independent research firm's report

D) a magazine advertisement for soap

Themes

Literary texts give concrete form to abstract, thematic ideas. Through a process of carefully examining the concrete details of a text and making evidence-based inferences, readers can come to understand the **theme** of a literary work—the universal message that authors hope to communicate through their artistic choices.

By tracing themes across time, location, and culture, readers can begin to recognize some of the common experiences that define humanity such as love, loss, power, betrayal, growing old, and coming of age.

To determine a theme, readers consider how authors craft their ideas using the literary tools of plot, setting, character, figurative language, and point of view. Through close reading and analysis of the author's choice, readers then infer what the author could be suggesting about life or human nature. Readers should

- ask focus questions to make connections with the text, like *how did the author's use of _____ affect your reaction to the story? Why would the author want you to react that way? What about this story can you relate to your own life?*;

- consider elements of the text, including the plot and character development, tone, setting, and figurative language;

- identify signal words or phrases, such as *as a result*, and consider their meaning.

By analyzing the author's purpose using specific details, readers can make connections, read more closely, and improve their critical reading and thinking skills.

PRACTICE QUESTION

19. What is the difference between the mood of a literary text and the author's tone?

    A) Readers experience the mood of a text; while reading, readers respond emotionally to the text and feel the mood. On the other hand, readers simply recognize the author's tone or attitude toward a subject as something that exists apart from them.

    B) Readers develop an understanding of how the characters feel, their moods, the attitudes they express, and their tone.

    C) The mood of a text is fluid; it changes as the characters develop. The tone of a text is stable; it is created by the words and symbols of the text.

    D) The mood of a text is understood at the end of a story and is created by how the conflict of the story is resolved. On the other hand, the reader recognizes the tone of a text right from the beginning.

Rhetorical Devices

In rhetoric, a deliberate effort is made to show the connection between points, to relate each point to the central idea, and to use words that will elicit a response from an audience.

To provide **rhetorical support** is to support generalizations, claims, and arguments with examples, details, and other evidence. Writers can support arguments by using the following:

- logical appeals (logos)

- emotional appeals (pathos)

- ethical appeals (ethos)

These rhetorical appeals are present in nearly all kinds of informative texts.

Figures of speech are expressions that are understood to have a nonliteral meaning. Writers use figurative language to suggest meaning, engage the reader's imagination, and add emphasis to different aspects of their subject.

TABLE 1.2. Figures of Speech and Rhetorical Devices		
DEVICE	**DEFINITION**	**EXAMPLE**
Metaphor	describes a topic as though it were something else more familiar	The car is the horse, and the driver is the jockey.
Simile	directly points to similarities between two things using comparative	I am as hungry as a horse.
Imagery	vivid description that appeals to the reader's sense of sight, sound, smell, taste, or touch	The big, shiny, dark brown horse stood tall as the wind blew through his mane, his hide shining in the sun.
Hyperbole	overstatement or exaggeration intended to achieve a particular effect	I am so hungry I could eat a horse!
Personification	human characteristics attributed to objects, abstract ideas, natural forces, or animals	The pine trees murmured in the breeze.
Symbolism	use of a concrete object, action, or character to represent an abstract idea	roses representing beauty, light representing truth, and darkness representing evil
Allusion	a reference to a historical person or event, a fictional character or event, a mythological or religious character or event, or an artist or artistic work	She had a Mona Lisa smile.
Cliché	common sayings that lack originality but are familiar and relatable to an audience	His question opened up a can of worms.
Dialect/Slang	linguistic qualities that indicate aspects about a character or make writing less formal	*y'all* versus *you all* *sneakers* versus *tennis shoes*
Foreshadowing	hinting at the events that are going to unfold in a story	Dorothy singing "Somewhere Over the Rainbow" before she lands in Oz
Verbal irony	when a character or narrator says something that is the opposite of what is meant	Someone who is having a bad day says, "I am having a great day!"

PRACTICE QUESTION

Alfie closed his eyes and took several deep breaths. He was trying to ignore the sounds of the crowd, but even he had to admit that it was hard not to notice the tension in the stadium. He could feel 50,000 sets of eyes burning through his skin—this crowd expected perfection from him. He took another breath and opened his eyes, setting his sights on the soccer ball resting peacefully in the grass. One shot, just one last shot, between his team and the championship. He didn't look up at the goalie, who was jumping nervously on the goal line just a few yards away. Afterward, he would swear he didn't remember anything between the referee's whistle and the thunderous roar of the crowd.

20. Which of the following best describes the meaning of the phrase "he could feel 50,000 sets of eyes burning through his skin"?

    A) The 50,000 people in the stadium are trying to hurt Alfie.

    B) Alfie feels uncomfortable and exposed in front of so many people.

    C) Alfie feels immense pressure from the 50,000 people watching him.

    D) The people in the stadium are warning Alfie that the field is on fire.

Vocabulary

On the Reading section you may also be asked to provide definitions or intended meanings of words within passages. You may have never encountered some of these words before the test, but there are tricks you can use to figure out what they mean.

Context Clues

One of the most fundamental vocabulary skills is using the context in which a word is found to determine its meaning. Your ability to read sentences carefully is extremely helpful when it comes to understanding new vocabulary words.

Vocabulary questions on the ATI TEAS will usually include **sentence context clues** within the sentence that contains the word. There are several clues that can help you understand the context and therefore the meaning of a word.

Restatement clues state the definition of the word in the sentence. The definition is often set apart from the rest of the sentence by a comma, parentheses, or a colon.

Teachers often prefer teaching students with <u>intrinsic</u> motivation: these students have an <u>internal</u> desire to learn.

The meaning of *intrinsic* is restated as *internal*.

Contrast clues include the opposite meaning of a word. Terms like *but, on the other hand*, and *however* are tip-offs that a sentence contains a contrast clue.

Janet was <u>destitute</u> after she lost her job, but her <u>wealthy</u> sister helped her get back on her feet.

> *Destitute* is contrasted with *wealthy*, so the
> definition of destitute is *poor*.

Positive/negative clues tell you whether a word has a positive or negative meaning.

> The film was <u>lauded</u> by critics as <u>stunning</u>, and was <u>nominated for several awards.</u>

> The positive descriptions *stunning* and *nominated for several awards* suggest that *lauded* has a positive meaning.

PRACTICE QUESTIONS

Select the answer that most closely matches the definition of the underlined word as it is used in the sentence.

21   The dog was <u>dauntless</u> in the face of danger, braving the fire to save the girl trapped inside the building.

A) difficult

B) fearless

C) imaginative

D) startled

22.   Beth did not spend any time preparing for the test, but Tyrone kept a <u>rigorous</u> study schedule.

A) strict

B) loose

C) boring

D) strange

 HELPFUL HINT

When answering vocabulary questions, try plugging each answer choice into the sentence to see if it makes sense.

Analyzing Words

As you know, determining the meaning of a word can be more complicated than just looking in a dictionary. A word might have more than one **denotation**, or definition, and which one the author intends can only be judged by looking at the surrounding text. For example, the word *quack* can refer to the sound a duck makes or to a person who publicly pretends to have a qualification they do not actually possess.

A word may also have different **connotations**, which are the implied meanings and emotions a word evokes in the reader. For example, a cubicle is simply a walled desk in an office, but for many the word implies a constrictive, uninspiring workplace. Connotations can vary greatly between cultures and even between individuals.

Authors might also employ **figurative language**, which uses a word to imply something other than the word's literal definition. This is often done by comparing two things. If you say, "I felt like a butterfly when I got a new haircut," the listener knows you do not resemble an insect but instead feel beautiful and transformed.

PRACTICE QUESTIONS

Select the answer that most closely matches the definition of the underlined word or phrase as it is used in the sentence.

23. The patient's uneven <u>pupils</u> suggested that brain damage was possible.

   A) part of the eye

   B) student in a classroom

   C) walking pace

   D) breathing sounds

24. Aiden examined the antique lamp and worried that he had been <u>taken for a ride</u>. He had paid a lot for the vintage lamp, but it looked like it was worthless.

   A) transported

   B) forgotten

   C) deceived

   D) hindered

Word Structure

You are not expected to know every word in the English language for your test; rather, you will need to use deductive reasoning to find the best definition of the word in question. Many words can be broken down into three main parts to help determine their meaning:

prefix – root – suffix

Roots are the building blocks of all words. Every word is either a root itself or has a root. The root is what is left when you strip away the prefixes and suffixes from a word. For example, if you take away the prefix *un–* from the word *unclear*, you have the root *clear*.

Roots are not always recognizable words because they often come from Latin or Greek words, such as *nat*, a Latin root meaning "born." The word *native*, which refers to a person born in a referenced place, comes from this root. So does the word *prenatal*, meaning "before birth." It is important to keep in mind, however, that roots do not always match the original definitions of words, and they can have several different spellings.

Prefixes are elements added to the beginning of a word, and **suffixes** are elements added to the end of a word; together they are known as affixes. They carry assigned meanings and can be attached to a word to completely change the word's meaning or to enhance the word's original meaning.

Let's use the word *prefix* itself as an example: *fix* means "to place something securely," and *pre–* means "before." Therefore, *prefix* means "to place something before or in front of." Now let's look at a suffix: in the word *feminism, femin* is

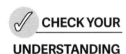

CHECK YOUR UNDERSTANDING

Can you figure out the definitions of the following words using their parts?

ambidextrous, anthropology, diagram, egocentric, hemisphere, homicide, metamorphosis, nonsense, portable, rewind, submarine, triangle, unicycle

a root that means "female." The suffix *–ism* means "act," "practice," or "process." Thus, *feminism* is the process of establishing equal rights for women.

Although you cannot determine the meaning of a word from a prefix or suffix alone, you can use this knowledge to eliminate answer choices. Understanding whether the word is positive or negative can give you the partial meaning of the word.

TABLE 1.3. Common Roots

ROOT	DEFINITION	EXAMPLE
ast(er)	star	asteroid, astronomy
audi	hear	audience, audible
auto	self	automatic, autograph
bene	good	beneficent, benign
bio	life	biology, biorhythm
cap	take	capture
ced	yield	secede
chrono	time	chronometer, chronic
corp	body	corporeal
crac or crat	rule	autocrat
demo	people	democracy
dict	say	dictionary, dictation
duc	lead or make	ductile, produce
gen	give birth	generation, genetics
geo	earth	geography, geometry
grad	step	graduate
graph	write	graphical, autograph
ject	throw	eject
jur or jus	law	justice, jurisdiction
juven	young	juvenile
log or logue	thought	logic, logarithm
luc	light	lucidity
man	hand	manual
mand	order	remand
mis	send	transmission
mono	one	monotone

continued on next page

TABLE 1.3. Common Roots (continued)

ROOT	DEFINITION	EXAMPLE
omni	all	omnivore
path	feel	sympathy
phil	love	philanthropy
phon	sound	phonograph
port	carry	export
qui	rest	quiet
scrib or script	write	scribe, transcript
sense or sent	feel	sentiment
tele	far away	telephone
terr	earth	terrace
uni	single	unicode
vac	empty	vacant
vid or vis	see	video, vision

TABLE 1.4. Common Prefixes

PREFIX	DEFINITION	EXAMPLE
a– (also an–)	not, without; to, toward; of, completely	atheist, anemic, aside, aback, anew, abashed
ante–	before, preceding	antecedent, anteroom
anti–	opposing, against	antibiotic, anticlimax
belli–	warlike, combative	belligerent, antebellum
com– (also co–, col–, con–, cor–)	with, jointly, completely	combat, cooperate, collide, confide, correspond
dis– (also di–)	negation, removal	disadvantage, disbar
en– (also em–)	put into or on; bring into the condition of; intensify	engulf, embrace
hypo–	under	hypoglycemic, hypodermic
in– (also il–, im–, ir–)	not, without; in, into, toward, inside	infertile, impossible, illegal, irregular, influence, include
intra–	inside, within	intravenous, intrapersonal
out–	surpassing, exceeding; external, away from	outperform, outdoor
over–	excessively, completely; upper, outer, over, above	overconfident, overcast

pre–	before	precondition, preadolescent, prelude
re–	again	reapply, remake
semi–	half, partly	semicircle, semiconscious
syn– (also sym–)	in union, acting together	synthesis, symbiotic
trans–	across, beyond	transdermal
trans–	into a different state	translate
under–	beneath, below; not enough	underarm, undersecretary, underdeveloped

PRACTICE QUESTIONS

Select the answer that most closely matches the definition of the underlined word as it is used in the sentence.

25. The <u>bellicose</u> dog will be sent to training school next week.

A) misbehaved

B) friendly

C) scared

D) aggressive

26. The new menu <u>rejuvenated</u> the restaurant and made it one of the most popular spots in town.

A) established

B) invigorated

C) improved

D) motivated

1. **B)** The topic of the passage is geysers. Tourists, volcanic eruptions, and supervolcanoes are all mentioned in the explanation of what geysers are and how they are formed.

2. **D)** The author writes, "the allied tribes of the Plains Indians decisively defeated their US foes," and the remainder of the passage provides details to support this idea. Choice A is a fact stated in the passage but is not general enough to be the main idea. Similarly, Choice C can be inferred from the passage, but it is not what the majority of the passage is about. Choice B is too general and discusses topics outside the content of the passage.

3. **B)** Choice B is the first sentence of the passage and introduces the topic. Choice A is the final sentence of the passage and summarizes the passage's content. Choices C and D are supporting sentences found within the body of the passage. They include important details that support the main idea.

4. **A)** The passage states, "The topography of Venus, for example, has been explored by several space probes, including the Russian Venera landers and NASA's *Magellan* orbiter." The other choices are mentioned in the passage but are not space probes.

5. **B)** Choice B is the best option because it supports the author's point about using multiple technologies to study the surface of planets. Choices C and D can be eliminated because they do not address the study of the surface of planets. Choice A can also be eliminated because it only addresses a single technology.

6. **B)** This placement fits with the paragraph's chronological order. The 1940s precede the 1950s, so the new sentence should precede sentence number two. The signal word *first* shows that sentence one should start the paragraph. The signal word *finally* in sentence three indicates that it is the final sentence, ruling out option D.

7. **B)** Starting with three red apples and one green apple, and following the directions, the basket will have
    1. two red apples and one green apple;
    2. two red apples and two green apples;
    3. three red apples and two green apples;
    4. three red apples and three green apples;
    5. one red apple and three green apples;
    6. one red apple and two green apples;
    7. four red apples and two green apples;
    8. four red apples and four green apples.

8. **C)** Starting with 12 gallons, and following the directions, the tank will have
   1. eleven gallons;
   2. ten gallons;
   3. nine and a half gallons;
   4. nine gallons;
   5. seven gallons.

9. **A)** According to the index, this information can be found on pages 237 – 291.

10. **C)** According to the table of contents, page 125 is in "Chapter 3: Geometry."

11. **C)** The sentence in choice C italicizes the title of a long work and is therefore correct. Italics are not used for names of cities and states (choice A), foods (choice B), or streets (choice D).

12. **B)** The purpose of the passage is to persuade the reader of the author's opinion of the novel *Mockingjay*, specifically that the ending did not do the main character justice. The author's use of the verb *argue* tells us that the passage is presenting a case to the reader. The passage follows this statement with evidence—that the main character had a powerful personality.

13. **A)** The passage is telling a story—we meet Elizabeth and learn about her fear of flying—so it is a narrative text. There is no factual information presented or explained, nor is the author trying to persuade the reader of anything.

14. **D)** Choice C is wrong because the author provides no root cause or a list of effects. Choices A and B are tricky, because the passage does compare two things (northern and southern cities) and describes a place (a sprawling city). However, the passage starts by presenting a problem (transportation) and then suggests a solution (trains and buses), making choice D the only one that addresses the organization of the entire passage.

15. **C)** In this text, a narrator is explaining facts about empathy using the third person ("it is the ability to actually share...")

16. **B)** Since the author argues that children need a proper diet rich in fruits and vegetables, we can infer that they would probably agree with choice B. The author describes the cost of health care as a problem for all Americans, implying that adults who never learned healthy eating habits should not be punished (choice A). Choices C and D are contradicted by the author's focus on creating healthy habits in schools.

17. **C)** Choice C is the only secondary source listed. Choices A, B, and D all contain firsthand information.

18. **C)** All four sources might discuss the effectiveness of the soap in question, but choice C, an independent research firm, is the most credible because it is a professional firm not related to the manufacturer.

19. **A)** The mood of a text is felt by readers as they interact with the text whereas the tone is more of a reflection of how the author feels, usually communicated through specific diction.

20. **C)** The metaphor implies that Alfie feels pressure to perform well from the people watching him. There is no indication that he is threatened physically.

21. **B)** Demonstrating bravery in the face of danger would be fearless. The restatement clue *(braving)* tells the reader exactly what the word means.

22. **A)** The word *but* is a contrast clue that tells us that Tyrone studied in a different way from Beth. If Beth did not study hard, then Tyrone did. The best answer, therefore, is choice A.

23. **A)** Only choice A matches both the definition of the word and the context of the sentence. Choice B is an alternative definition for *pupil*, but it does not make sense in the sentence. Both choices C and D could be correct in the context of the sentence, but neither is a definition of *pupil*.

24. **C)** It is clear from the context of the sentence that Aiden was not literally taken for a ride. Instead, this phrase is an example of figurative language. From context clues you can figure out that Aiden paid too much for the lamp, so he was deceived.

25. **D)** Both *misbehaved* and *aggressive* look like possible answers given the context of the sentence. However, the prefix *belli–*, which means "warlike," can be used to confirm that *aggressive* is the correct answer.

26. **B)** All the answer choices could make sense in the context of the sentence, so it is necessary to use word structure to find the definition. The root *juven* means "young," and the prefix *re–* means "again," so *rejuvenate* means "to be made young again." The answer choice with the most similar meaning is *invigorated*, which means "to give something energy."

Reading Graphics

The ATI TEAS exam also includes questions that test your comprehension of informational sources other than text passages. These questions will include visual information sources (maps, graphs, diagrams), text features (book indexes, tables of contents), printed communications (flyers, memos), or lists of instructions.

Graphs

Graphs are used to present numerical data in a way that is easy for the reader to understand. There are a number of different types of graphs, each of which is useful for different types of data.

Bar graphs use bars of different lengths to compare amounts. The independent variable on a bar graph is grouped into categories like months, flavors, or locations, and the dependent variable is a quantity. Thus, comparing the lengths of the bars provides a visual guide to the relative quantities in each category.

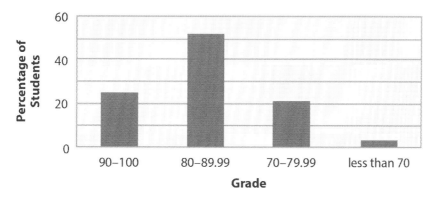

Figure 2.1. Bar Graph

Scatterplots use points to show relationships between two variables that can be plotted as coordinate points. One variable describes a position on the *x*-axis, and the other a point on the *y*-axis. Scatterplots can suggest relationships between variables. For example, both variables might increase, or one might increase when the other decreases.

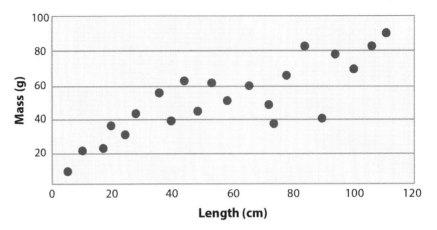

Figure 2.2. Scatterplot

Line graphs show changes in data by connecting points on a scatterplot using a line. These graphs will often measure time on the *x*-axis and are used to show trends in the data, such as temperature changes over a day or school attendance throughout the year.

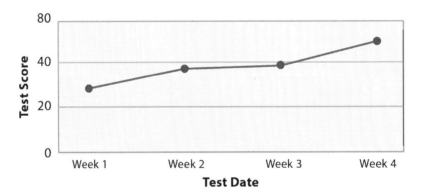

Figure 2.3. Line Graph

Circle graphs (also called pie charts) are used to show parts of a whole: the "pie" is the whole, and each "slice" represents a percentage or part of the whole.

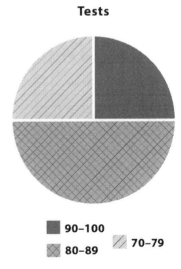

Figure 2.4. Circle Graph

PRACTICE QUESTIONS

1. Which of the following products accounts for the largest share of Wholesale Electronics' total sales?

Sales at Wholesale Electronics

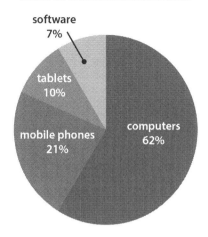

A) mobile phones

B) computers

C) software and tablets

D) software and mobile phones

2. Mobile phones and tablets make up what percentage of Wholesale Electronics' total sales?

A) 17 percent

B) 28 percent

C) 31 percent

D) 83 percent

Maps

The **legend**, or **key**, of a map explains the various symbols used on the map and their meanings and measurements. These symbols typically include a compass rose and a distance scale. A **compass rose** indicates the four cardinal directions (north, south, west, and east) and the four intermediate directions (northwest, northeast, southwest, and southeast). A **distance scale** is used to show the ratio of the distance on the page to the actual distance between objects, usually in miles or kilometers.

→
CONTINUE

PRACTICE QUESTIONS

3. Which direction is Ruby Stone Lake from Park Headquarters?

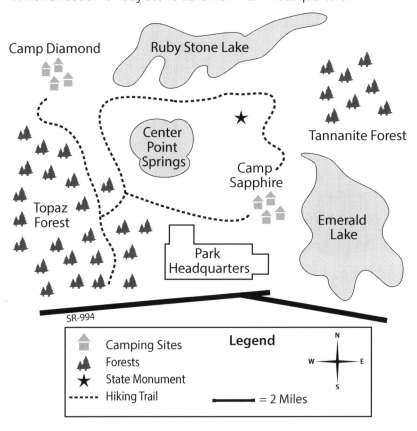

A) south

B) northwest

C) southwest

D) north

4. Approximately how many miles is it from the state monument to the center of Tannanite Forest?

A) 1 mile

B) 2 miles

C) 4 miles

D) 5 miles

Scale Readings

A **scale reading** is a numerical value collected from a scale or measurement device. Some questions on the TEAS may refer to devices like thermometers, blood pressure cuffs, or weight scales. To prepare for the exam, familiarize yourself with the standard units and displays for these devices.

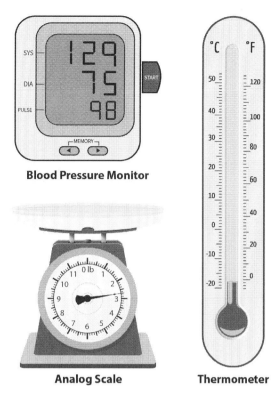

Blood Pressure Monitor

Analog Scale

Thermometer

Figure 2.5. Scale Readings

PRACTICE QUESTIONS

5. The figure shows the readout for a patient's EKG monitor. What is the patient's oxygen saturation?

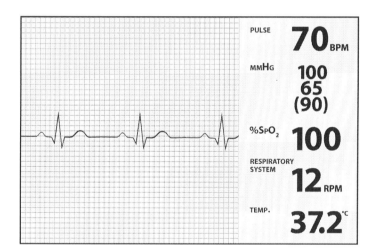

A) 70 BPM

B) 100 mmHg

C) 100 percent

D) 37.2°C

CONTINUE

The table below describes the categories for systolic blood pressure.

Categories	Systolic Range
Normal	< 120
Prehypertension	120 – 139
Hypertension Stage 1	140 – 159
Hypertension Stage 2	160 – 179
Hypertensive Crisis	> 180

6. The EKG monitor shows a patient who belongs in which of the following categories?

    A) Normal

    B) Prehypertension

    C) Hypertension Stage 1

    D) Hypertension Stage 2

Product Information

Product information questions ask you to use given information about products, such as price, shipping, or taxes, to compare the true cost of those products. (You will be required to perform basic arithmetic for some of the problems in this section.)

PRACTICE QUESTIONS

Use the chart below to answer the following questions.

Shoe Prices			
RETAILER	BASE PRICE	SHIPPING & HANDLING	TAXES
Wholesale Footwear	$59.99	$10.95	$7.68
Bargain Sales	$65.99	$5.95	$5.38
Famous Shoes	$79.99	$0.00	$4.89

7. Rachel wants to buy shoes and can't spend more than $80. Which retailer(s) can she shop at?

    A) Wholesale Footwear and Bargain Sales

    B) Famous Shoes

    C) Wholesale Footwear and Famous Shoes

    D) Bargain Sales and Famous Shoes

8. Allen has budgeted $6 for taxes and $6 for shipping and handling. Which retailer(s) can he shop at?

    A) Bargain Sales and Famous Shoes

    B) Wholesale Footwear and Famous Shoes

    C) Wholesale Footwear

    D) Bargain Sales and Wholesale Footwear

Using Graphics

In some texts, graphics—pictures, diagrams, graphs, and other figures—are used to strengthen arguments. Graphics can provide supporting evidence for a piece of writing, further illustrate a point, or engage the reader.

Take, for example, the following passage:

> The consumer price index (CPI) measures prices of goods and services as they change over time. Economists select a "base year" and compile a market "basket" of 400 consumer goods and services (like gas, appliances, and groceries) from that year. They create the price index by measuring the change in prices. Over the years, prices have increased in the United States.
>
> The graph below shows a sample of the CPI in the United States between 1913 and 2010. The dark line shows the average CPI for each year, with 1982 – 1984 as the "base year" (when CPI = 100). The numbers on the left represent the CPI, ranging from 0 to 250. The percentages on the right represent levels of increase or decrease beyond the CPI of the base year.
>
> The light line ("Change in Average Consumer Price Index") represents the percent change in average CPI from year to year.

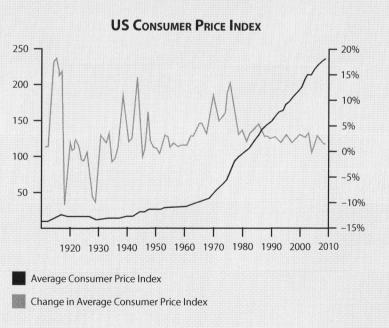

US Consumer Price Index

■ Average Consumer Price Index

■ Change in Average Consumer Price Index

Plenty of information is available in this passage. But providing a graph helps the reader visualize the text. The sharp increase in prices from 1970 onward helps prove the writer's argument that prices have increased.

Still, even visual aids can be misleading. It is important to critically analyze graphics to uncover any biased or misleading information.

For example, in the CPI graph, it is not possible to determine whether the prices of specific goods increased or decreased. The graph only reflects the "basket" of 400 goods. Certain items, like gasoline, fluctuate widely in price. Just because the CPI increased since 1970 does not mean that the prices of *all* goods rose and have stayed high.

Furthermore, the graphic does not consider economic phenomena like globalization or wage increases. Certain items that were out of reach for most Americans in the early twentieth century (like automobiles, electronics, and single-family homes) are now more available in the early twenty-first century thanks to credit, cheaper prices due to overseas manufacturing, and social change.

PRACTICE QUESTION

Using the text and graph above, answer the following question about CPI.

9. According to the graph, how has the Average Consumer Price Index changed over time?

   A) It has remained constant.

   B) It has fluctuated, stabilizing toward the end of the century and the early 2000s.

   C) It was stable in the early twentieth century, but it became unstable in the early 2000s.

   D) It has been unstable since the early twentieth century.

1. **B)** Computers account for 62 percent of sales. Mobile phones (choice A) are 21 percent, software and tablets (choice C) equal 17 percent, and software and mobile phones (choice D) equal 28 percent.

2. **C)** Mobile phones (21 percent) and tablets (10 percent) together account for 31 percent of Wholesale Electronics' total sales.

3. **D)** Ruby Stone Lake is north of Park Headquarters.

4. **C)** Using the distance scale, it is possible to estimate that the center of Tannanite Forest is approximately 4 miles from the state monument.

5. **C)** The notation %SpO$_2$ stands for oxygen saturation, which reads 100 percent.

6. **A)** The EKG monitor shows a systolic reading of 100, which places the patient in the Normal category.

7. **A)** When you add the base price, shipping and handling fees, and taxes, shoes from Famous Shoes cost $84.88, so Rachel can only shop at Wholesale Footwear ($78.62) and Bargain Sales ($77.32).

8. **A)** Bargain Sales and Famous Shoes are both under Allen's budget for taxes and shipping and handling.

9. **B)** The gray line that depicts change in average CPI fluctuates in the early twentieth century, swinging to a high of 250 then dropping below 50—all before 1920. Throughout the 1920s, the average swings from just above 100 to below 50. In the 1940s, it swings from 100 to above 200. However, from the 1980s onward, the line is mostly stable, aside from a dip after the year 2000.

PART

2 | Mathematics

The ATI TEAS Mathematics test covers mathematical concepts studied in high school. These concepts are broken down into four categories.

Numbers: basic arithmetic operations, exponents and radicals, fractions, ratios, percents

- Algebra: expressions, equations, inequalities, graphing on a coordinate plane

- Measurement: units, geometric shapes, perimeter, area, volume

- Data: statistics, graphs

You will be provided a drop-down four-function calculator on the computer version of the TEAS, so you don't need to worry about being able to perform basic calculations on your own. Instead, the test will focus on your understanding of mathematical concepts and relationships.

Numbers and Operations

Arithmetic Operations

The four basic arithmetic operations are addition, subtraction, multiplication, and division.

- **Add** to combine two or more quantities ($6 + 5 = 11$).
- **Subtract** to find the difference of two or more quantities ($10 - 3 = 7$).
- **Multiply** to add a quantity multiple times ($4 \times 3 = 12 \Leftrightarrow 3 + 3 + 3 + 3 = 12$).
- **Divide** to determine how many times one quantity goes into another ($10 \div 2 = 5$).

Word problems contain **clue words** that help you determine which operation to use.

TABLE 3.1. Operations Word Problems		
OPERATION	**CLUE WORDS**	**EXAMPLE**
Addition	sum together (in) total all in addition increased give	Leslie has 3 pencils. If her teacher **gives** her 2 pencils, how many does she now have **in total**? $3 + 2 = 5$ pencils
Subtraction	minus less than take (away) decreased difference How many left? How many more/less?	Sean has 12 cookies. His sister **takes** 2 cookies. **How many** cookies does Sean have **left**? $12 - 2 = 10$ cookies

CONTINUE →

TABLE 3.1. Operations Word Problems (continued)

OPERATION	CLUE WORDS	EXAMPLE
Multiplication	product times of each/every groups of twice	A hospital department has 10 patient rooms. If **each** room holds 2 patients, how many patients can stay in the department? $10 \times 2 = 20$ patients
Division	divided per each/every distributed average How many for each? How many groups?	A teacher has 150 stickers to **distribute** to her class of 25 students. If each student gets the same number of stickers, **how many** stickers will **each** student get? $150 \div 25 = 6$ stickers

PRACTICE QUESTION

1. A case of pencils contains 10 boxes. Each box contains 150 pencils. How many pencils are in the case?

    A) 15

    B) 160

    C) 1500

    D) 16,000

Exponents and Radicals

Exponential expressions, such as 5^3, contain a base and an exponent. The **exponent** indicates how many times to use the **base** as a factor. In the expression 5^3, 5 is the base and 3 is the exponent. The value of 5^3 is found by multiplying 5 by itself three times: $5^3 = 5 \times 5 \times 5 = 125$. Rules for working with exponents are given in the table below.

TABLE 3.2. Operations with Exponents

RULE	EXAMPLE
$a^0 = 1$	$5^0 = 1$
$a^{-n} = \frac{1}{a^n}$	$5^{-3} = \frac{1}{5^3}$
$a^m a^n = a^{m+n}$	$5^3 5^4 = 5^{3+4} = 5^7$
$(a^m)^n = a^{m \times n}$	$(5^3)^4 = 5^{3(4)} = 5^{12}$

RULE	EXAMPLE
$\dfrac{a^m}{a^n} = a^{m-n}$	$\dfrac{5^4}{5^3} = 5^{4-3} = 5^1$
$(ab)^n = a^n b^n$	$(5 \times 6)^3 = 5^3 6^3$
$\left(\dfrac{a}{b}\right)^n = \dfrac{a^n}{b^n}$	$\left(\dfrac{5}{6}\right)^3 = \dfrac{5^3}{6^3}$
$\left(\dfrac{a}{b}\right)^{-n} = \left(\dfrac{b}{a}\right)^n$	$\left(\dfrac{5}{6}\right)^{-3} = \left(\dfrac{6}{5}\right)^3$
$\dfrac{a^{-m}}{b^{-n}} = \dfrac{b^n}{a^m}$	$\dfrac{5^{-3}}{6^{-4}} = \dfrac{6^4}{5^3}$

Finding the **root** of a number is the inverse of raising a number to a power. In other words, the root is the number of times a value should be multiplied by itself to reach a given value. Roots are named for the power on the base:

- 5 is the **square root** of 25 because $5^2 = 25$
- 5 is the **cube root** of 125 because $5^3 = 125$
- 5 is the **fourth root** of 625, because $5^4 = 625$

The symbol for finding the root of a number is the radical: $\sqrt{\ }$. By itself, the radical indicates a square root: $\sqrt{36} = 6$ because $6^2 = 36$. Other numbers can be included in front of the radical to indicate different roots: $\sqrt[4]{1296} = 6$ because $6^4 = 1296$. Rules for working with radicals are given in the table below.

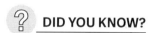 **DID YOU KNOW?**

The number under the radical is called the **radicand**.

TABLE 3.3. Operations with Radicals

RULE	EXAMPLE
$\sqrt[b]{ac} = \sqrt[b]{a}\,\sqrt[b]{c}$	$\sqrt[3]{81} = \sqrt[3]{27}\,\sqrt[3]{3} = 3\sqrt[3]{3}$
$\sqrt[b]{\dfrac{a}{c}} = \dfrac{\sqrt[b]{a}}{\sqrt[b]{c}}$	$\sqrt{\dfrac{4}{81}} = \dfrac{\sqrt{4}}{\sqrt{81}} = \dfrac{2}{9}$
$\sqrt[b]{a^c} = (\sqrt[b]{a})^c = a^{\frac{c}{b}}$	$\sqrt[3]{6^2} = (\sqrt[3]{6})^2 = 6^{\frac{2}{3}}$

PRACTICE QUESTIONS

2. Which of the following values is equivalent to $\sqrt{48}$?

   A) $16\sqrt{3}$

   B) $4\sqrt{3}$

   C) $3\sqrt{4}$

   D) $2\sqrt{12}$

3. Which of the following values is the smallest?

   $2^0, 2^{1/2}, 2^{-2}, 2^1$

   A) 2^0

   B) $2^{1/2}$

   C) 2^{-2}

   D) 2^1

Order of Operations

Operations in a mathematical expression are always performed in a specific order, which is described by the acronym PEMDAS:

1. Parentheses
2. Exponents
3. Multiplication
4. Division
5. Addition
6. Subtraction

Perform the operations within parentheses first, and then address any exponents. After those steps, perform all multiplication and division. These are carried out from left to right as they appear in the problem. Finally, do all required addition and subtraction, also from left to right as each operation appears in the problem.

Simplify the expression $(3^2 - 2)^2 + (4)5^3$.

Parentheses	$(3^2 - 2)^2 + (4)5^3$ $= (9 - 2)^2 + (4)5^3$ $= 7^2 + (4)5^3$
Exponents	$= 49 + (4)125$
Multiplication and division	$= 49 + 500$
Addition and subtraction	$= 549$

PRACTICE QUESTIONS

4. Simplify: $15 \times (4 + 8) - 33$

   A) −1500

   B) −315

   C) 35

   D) 147

5. Simplify: $-(3)^2 + 4(5) + (5 - 6)^2 - 8$

   A) 2

   B) 4

   C) 22

   D) 29

Fractions

A **fraction** represents parts of a whole. The top number of a fraction, called the **numerator**, indicates how many equal-sized parts are present. The bottom number of a fraction, called the **denominator**, indicates how many equal-sized parts make a whole.

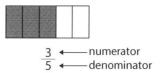

$$\frac{3}{5} \leftarrow \text{numerator} \atop \leftarrow \text{denominator}$$

Figure 3.1. Parts of Fractions

Fractions have several forms:

- **proper fraction**: the numerator is less than the denominator
- **improper fraction**: the numerator is greater than or equal to the denominator
- **mixed number**: the combination of a whole number and a fraction

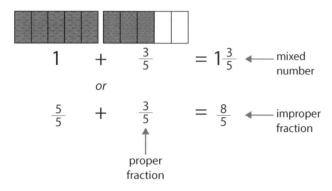

Figure 3.2. Types of Fractions

Improper fractions can be converted to mixed numbers by dividing. In fact, the fraction bar is also a division symbol.

$$\tfrac{14}{3} = 14 \div 3 = 4 \text{ (with 2 left over)} = 4\tfrac{2}{3}$$

To convert a mixed number to a fraction, multiply the whole number by the denominator of the fraction, and add the numerator. The result becomes the numerator of the improper fraction; the denominator remains the same.

$$5\tfrac{2}{3} = \frac{(5 \times 3) + 2}{3} = \frac{17}{3}$$

To **multiply fractions**, multiply numerators and multiply denominators. Reduce the product to lowest terms. To **divide fractions**, multiply the first fraction by the reciprocal of the second fraction. When multiplying and dividing mixed numbers, the mixed numbers must be converted to improper fractions.

$$\frac{a}{b} \times \frac{c}{d} = \frac{ac}{bd}$$

$$\frac{a}{b} \div \frac{c}{d} = \left(\frac{a}{b}\right)\left(\frac{d}{c}\right) = \frac{ad}{bc}$$

 HELPFUL HINT

The **reciprocal** of a fraction is just the fraction with the top and bottom numbers switched.

Adding or subtracting fractions requires a common denominator. To find a **common denominator**, multiply the denominators of the fractions. Then, to add the fractions, add the numerators and keep the denominator the same.

$$\frac{a}{b} + \frac{c}{b} = \frac{a+c}{b}$$

$$\frac{a}{b} - \frac{c}{b} = \frac{a-c}{b}$$

PRACTICE QUESTIONS

6. Which of the following quantities is the greatest?

    A) $2\frac{3}{4}$

    B) $\frac{26}{16}$

    C) $3\frac{1}{2}$

    D) $\frac{35}{8}$

7. Ari and Teagan each ordered a pizza. Ari has $\frac{1}{4}$ of his pizza left, and Teagan has $\frac{1}{3}$ of her pizza left. How much total pizza do they have left?

    A) $\frac{1}{2}$ pizza

    B) $\frac{2}{7}$ pizza

    C) $\frac{7}{12}$ pizza

    D) $\frac{3}{4}$ pizza

Decimals

Numbers are written using the base-10 system, where each digit (the numeric symbols 0 – 9) in a number is worth ten times as much as the number to the right of it. For example, in the number 37 each digit has a place value based on its location. The 3 is in the tens place, and so has a value of 30, and the 7 is in the ones place, so it has a value of 7.

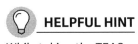

HELPFUL HINT

While taking the TEAS, you'll be able to use a calculator to perform operations with decimals.

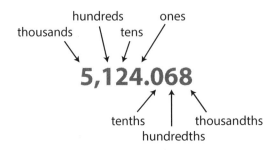

Figure 3.3. Place Value

Converting Decimals to Fractions

To convert a decimal, use the numbers that come after the decimal as the numerator in the fraction. The denominator will be a power of 10 that matches the place value for the original decimal. For example, the denominator for 0.46 would be 100 because the last number is in the hundredths place; likewise, the denominator for 0.657 would be 1000 because the last number is in the thousandths place. Once this fraction has been set up, all that's left is to simplify it.

$$2.375 = 2 + \tfrac{375}{1000} = 2 + \tfrac{3(125)}{8(125)} = 2 + \tfrac{3}{8} = 2\tfrac{3}{8}$$

PRACTICE QUESTION

8. Which of the following numbers is equivalent to 0.45?

A) $\dfrac{9}{100}$

B) $\dfrac{46}{100}$

C) $\dfrac{9}{20}$

D) $\dfrac{4}{5}$

DID YOU KNOW?

To convert a fraction to a decimal, just divide the numerator by the denominator on your calculator.

Scientific Notation

Scientific notation is a method of representing very large and very small numbers in the form $a \times 10^n$, where a is a value between 1 and 10, and n is a nonzero integer. For example, the number 927,000,000 is written in scientific notation as 9.27×10^8. The rules of exponents are used to perform operations with numbers in scientific notation.

- When adding and subtracting numbers in scientific notation, write all numbers with the same n value and add or subtract the a values.

- When multiplying numbers in scientific notation, multiply the a values and add the n values (exponents).

- To divide numbers in scientific notation, divide the a values and subtract the n values (exponents).

PRACTICE QUESTION

9. Which of the following shows the expression $(3.8 \times 10^3) + (4.7 \times 10^2)$ written correctly in scientific notation?

A) 42.7×10^2

B) 4.27×10^3

C) 85×10^4

D) 8.5×10^5

Comparison of Rational Numbers

Number comparison problems present numbers in different formats and ask which is larger or smaller, or whether the numbers are equivalent. The important step in solving these problems is to convert the numbers to the same format so that it is easier to see how they compare. If numbers are given in the same format, or after they have been converted, determine which number is smaller or if the numbers are equal. Remember that for negative numbers, higher numbers are actually smaller.

> Order the numbers from least to greatest:
> $$\frac{3}{8}, -0.75, -1\frac{3}{5}, \frac{5}{4}, 0.6, \text{ and } -0.2$$
>
> Convert each fraction to a decimal:
> $$\frac{3}{8} = 0.375, -1\frac{3}{5} = -1.6, \text{ and } \frac{5}{4} = 1.25$$
>
> Plot each decimal value on a number line.
>
>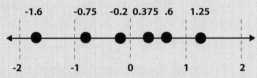
>
> Order from least to greatest (left to right on the number line) using the original given values.
> $$-1\frac{3}{5}, -0.75, -0.2, \frac{3}{8}, 0.6, \text{ and } \frac{5}{4}$$

PRACTICE QUESTION

10. Place the following numbers in order from least to greatest:

$\frac{2}{5}, -0.7, 0.35, -\frac{3}{2}, 0.46$

A) $-\frac{3}{2} < -0.7 < 0.35 < \frac{2}{5} < 0.46$

B) $-0.7 < -\frac{3}{2} < \frac{2}{5} < 0.35 < 0.46$

C) $-\frac{3}{2} < -0.7 < \frac{2}{5} < 0.35 < 0.46$

D) $-0.7 < -\frac{3}{2} < 0.35 < \frac{2}{5} < 0.46$

Ratios and Proportions

A **ratio** is a comparison of two quantities. For example, if a class consists of 15 women and 10 men, the ratio of women to men is 15 to 10. This ratio can also be written as 15:10 or $\frac{15}{10}$. Ratios, like fractions, can be reduced by dividing by common factors.

A **proportion** is a statement that two ratios are equal. For example, the proportion $\frac{5}{10} = \frac{7}{14}$ is true because both ratios are equal to $\frac{1}{2}$. The cross product is found by multiplying the numerator of one fraction by the denominator of the other (*across* the equal sign):

$$\frac{a}{b} = \frac{c}{d} \rightarrow ad = bc$$

The fact that the cross products of proportions are equal can be used to solve proportions in which one of the values is missing. Use x to represent the missing value, then cross multiply and solve.

$$\frac{5}{x} = \frac{7}{14}$$

$$5(14) = x(7)$$

$$70 = 7x$$

$$x = 10$$

One last important thing to consider when working with ratios is the units of the values being compared. On the TEAS, you may be asked to rewrite a ratio using the same units on both sides. For example, you might have to rewrite the ratio "3 minutes to 7 seconds" as "180 seconds to 7 seconds."

PRACTICE QUESTIONS

11. In a theater, there are 4500 lower-level seats and 2000 upper-level seats. What is the ratio of lower-level seats to total seats?

 A) $\frac{4}{13}$

 B) $\frac{4}{9}$

 C) $\frac{9}{13}$

 D) $\frac{9}{4}$

12. The dosage for a particular medication is proportional to the weight of the patient. If the dosage for a patient weighing 60 kg is 90 mg, what is the dosage for a patient weighing 80 kg?

 A) 53.3 mg

 B) 68 mg

 C) 106.7 mg

 D) 120 mg

Percents

A **percent** (or percentage) means *per hundred* and is written with the symbol %. For example, 36% means 36 out of 100. A percent can be turned into a decimal by moving the decimal point two places to the left (i.e., dividing by 100): 36% = 0.36. Percentages can be solved by setting up a proportion:

$$\frac{\text{part}}{\text{whole}} = \frac{\%}{100}$$

Percent change describes how much a given quantity has changed. The problems are solved in a similar way to regular percent problems using these formulas:

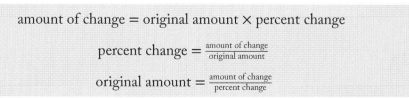

$$\text{amount of change} = \text{original amount} \times \text{percent change}$$

$$\text{percent change} = \frac{\text{amount of change}}{\text{original amount}}$$

$$\text{original amount} = \frac{\text{amount of change}}{\text{percent change}}$$

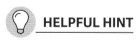

HELPFUL HINT

Words that indicate a percent change problem include *discount, markup, sale, increase,* and *decrease.*

13. On Tuesday, a radiology clinic had 80% of patients come in for their scheduled appointments. If they saw 16 patients, how many scheduled appointments did the clinic have on Tuesday?

A) 11

B) 12

C) 20

D) 22

14. A smart HDTV that originally cost $1,500 is on sale for 45% off. What is the sale price for the item?

A) $675

B) $825

C) $1,455

D) $2,727

15. Kevin is planning a party and can host 120 people. If he sends out invitations to his friends and expects 30% to decline, what is the maximum number of invitations he should send?

A) 36

B) 84

C) 171

D) 400

Estimation and Rounding

Rounding is used to make numbers easier to work with. While the process makes numbers less accurate, it makes operations and mental math easier. Rounding is performed to a specific place value, such as the thousands or tenths place.

To round a number, first identify the digit in the specified place (such as the tens or hundreds). Then look at the digit one place to the right. If that digit is four or less, keep the digit in the specified place the same. If that digit is five or more, add 1 to the digit in the specified place. All the digits to the right of the specified place become zeros.

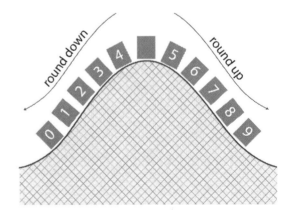

Figure 3.4. Rounding

rounded to the hundreds place: 5,372 → 5,400
rounded to the tens place: 5,372 → 5,370
rounded to the tenths place: 11.635 → 11.600
rounded to the hundredths place: 11.635 → 11.640

Estimation is when numbers are rounded and then an operation is performed. This process can be used when working with large numbers to find a close, but not exact, answer.

PRACTICE QUESTIONS

16. The populations of five local towns are given below:

TOWN	POPULATION
A	12,341
B	8,975
C	9,431
D	10,521
E	11,627

Which of the following values is closest to the total population of the five towns?

A) 50,000

B) 53,000

C) 55,000

D) 58,000

1. **C)** Multiply the number of boxes by the number of pencils in each box to find the total number of pencils:

   $10 \times 150 =$ **1500 pencils**

2. **B)** Determine the largest square number that is a factor of the radicand 48. Write the radicand as a product using that square number as a factor.

   $\sqrt{48} = \sqrt{16 \times 3} = \sqrt{16}\sqrt{3} =$ **$4\sqrt{3}$**

3. **C)**

   A: $2^0 = 1$

   B: $2^{1/2} = \sqrt{2} \approx 1.4$

   C: $\mathbf{2^{-2} = \frac{1}{2^2} = \frac{1}{4}}$

   D: $2^1 = 2$

4. **D)**

   $15 \times (4 + 8) - 33$

   $= 15 \times 12 - 33$

   $= 180 - 33$

   $= \mathbf{147}$

5. **B)**

   $-(3)^2 + 4(5) + (5 - 6)^2 - 8$

   $= -(3)^2 + 4(5) + (-1)^2 - 8$

   $= -9 + 4(5) + 1 - 8$

   $= -9 + 20 + 1 - 8$

   $= 11 + 1 - 8$

   $= 12 - 8$

   $= \mathbf{4}$

6. **D)** Write each number as an improper fraction with a common denominator:

   A: $2\frac{3}{4} = \frac{(2 \times 4) + 3}{4} = \frac{11}{4}\left(\frac{22}{2}\right) = \frac{22}{8}$

   B: $\frac{26}{16} = \frac{13(2)}{8(2)} = \frac{13}{8}$

   C: $3\frac{1}{2} = \frac{(3 \times 2) + 1}{2} = \frac{7}{2}\frac{4}{(4)} = \frac{28}{8}$

   D: $\mathbf{\frac{35}{8}}$

7. **C)** The common denominator is $4 \times 3 = 12$.

   Convert each fraction to the common denominator:

   $\frac{1}{4}\frac{3}{(3)} = \frac{3}{12}$

   $\frac{1}{3}\frac{4}{(4)} = \frac{4}{12}$

   Add the numerators and keep the denominator the same:

   $\frac{3}{12} + \frac{4}{12} = \frac{7}{12}$

   Together, they have $\frac{7}{12}$ of a pizza.

8. **C)**
$$0.45 = \frac{45}{100} = \frac{9(5)}{20(5)} = \frac{9}{20}$$

9. **B)** To add, the powers of 10 must be the same. Convert the first value so the power of 10 is 2:

$3.8 \times 10^3 = 3.8 \times 10 \times 10^2 = 38 \times 10^2$

Add the a terms together and write the answer in proper scientific notation, where $1 \leq a < 10$:

$(38 \times 10^2) + (4.7 \times 10^2) = (38 + 4.7) \times 10^2 = 42.7 \times 10^2 = \mathbf{4.27 \times 10^3}$

10. **A)** Convert the fractions to decimals:

$\frac{2}{5}$, -0.7, 0.35, $-\frac{3}{2}$, 0.46

$\frac{2}{5} = 0.4$

$-\frac{3}{2} = -1.5$

Place the values in order from smallest to largest:

$-1.5 < -0.7 < 0.35 < 0.4 < 0.46$

Put the numbers back in their original form:

$\mathbf{-\frac{3}{2} < -0.7 < 0.35 < \frac{2}{5} < 0.46}$

11. **C)** Total seats $= 4500 + 2000 = 6500$

$\frac{\text{lower seats}}{\text{total seats}} = \frac{4500}{6500} = \mathbf{\frac{9}{13}}$

12. **D)** Write a proportion using x for the missing value:

$$\frac{60 \text{ kg}}{90 \text{ mg}} = \frac{80 \text{ kg}}{x \text{ mg}}$$

Cross multiply:

$60(x) = 80(90)$

Divide by 60:

$60x = 7200$

$x = \mathbf{120 \text{ mg}}$

13. **C)** Set up a proportion and solve:

$$\frac{\text{part}}{\text{whole}} = \frac{\%}{100}$$

$$\frac{16}{x} = \frac{80}{100}$$

$16(100) = 80(x)$

$x = \mathbf{20}$

14. **B)** Identify the known values, then substitute in the percentage equation:

original amount $= \$1,500$

percent change $= 45\% = 0.45$

amount of change $= ?$

amount of change $=$ *original amount* $\times$ *percent change* $=$

$\$1,500 \times 0.45 = \$675$

Find the new price:

original price $-$ *amount of change* $=$ *new price*

$\$1,500 - \$675 = \mathbf{\$825}$

15. **C)** Kevin can only have 120 people attend. More than 120 people can be invited if he expects 30% to decline his invitation.
Convert percentage to decimal:
Accept invitation $\rightarrow$ 70% = 0.7
Let x = the number of people he can invite:
$x(0.7) = 120$
$x = \frac{120}{0.7}$
$x = \mathbf{171}$

16. **B)** Round each town population to the nearest thousand.
1$\underline{2}$,341 $\approx$ 12,000

$\underline{8}$,975 $\approx$ 9,000

$\underline{9}$,431 $\approx$ 9,000

1$\underline{0}$,521 $\approx$ 11,000

1$\underline{1}$,627 $\approx$ 12,000

Add to find the total population.

12,000 + 9,000 + 9,000 + 11,000 + 12,000 = **53,000**

4 | Algebra

Expressions and Equations

Algebraic expressions and equations include a **variable**, which is a letter standing in for a number. These expressions and equations are made up of **terms**, which are groups of numbers and variables (e.g., $2xy$). An **expression** is simply a set of terms (e.g., $3x + 2xy$). To evaluate an algebraic expression, plug in the given value(s) for the appropriate variable(s) in the expression.

> Find the value of $x^2 + 3$ when $x = 5$.
> $$x^2 + 3$$
> $$(5)^2 + 3 = 28$$

In an expression, only **like terms**—which have the exact same variable(s)—can be added or subtracted. **Constants** are numbers without variables attached, and those can be added and subtracted together as well. When simplifying an expression, like terms should be added or subtracted so that no individual group of variables occurs in more than one term.

> $2x + \underline{3xy} - 2z + 6y + \underline{2xy} \rightarrow 2x - 2z + 6y + (\underline{3xy} + \underline{2xy}) \rightarrow 2x - 2z + 6y + \underline{5xy}$

To multiply a single term by another, simply add the coefficients and then multiply the variables. Remember that when multiplying variables with exponents, those exponents are added together. For example, $(x^5 y)(x^3 y^4) = x^8 y^5$.

When multiplying a term by a set of terms inside parentheses, you need to **distribute** to each term inside the parentheses, as shown in Figure 4.1.

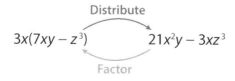

Figure 4.1. Distributing and Factoring

HELPFUL HINT

If the term outside the parentheses is negative, remember to distribute the negative to each term in the parentheses.

HELPFUL HINT

To multiply binomials (expressions with two terms), use FOIL: First – Outer – Inner – Last: $(a + b)(c + d) = ac + ad + bc + bd$.

When variables occur in both the numerator and the denominator of a fraction, they cancel each other out. So, a fraction with variables in its simplest form will not have the same variable on the top and bottom.

PRACTICE QUESTIONS

1. Evaluate the following expression for $a = -10$:

   $\frac{a^2}{4} - 3a + 4$

   A) −51

   B) −1

   C) 9

   D) 59

2. Evaluate the following expression for $a = xy$ and $b = x^2$:

   $2a + 3b$

   A) $2xy + 3x^2$

   B) $3xy + 2x^2$

   C) $5xy + 5x^2$

   D) $6x^3y$

3. Simplify the expression: $4x - 3y + 12z + 2x - 7y - 10z$

   A) $6x - 10y + 2z$

   B) $6x + 10y - 2z$

   C) $-2xyz$

   D) $-x + 14z - 17y$

4. Expand the following expression: $5x(x^2 - 2c + 10)$

   A) $5x^3 + 10xc + 50x$

   B) $5x^3 - 10xc + 50x$

   C) $5x^2 - 10c + 50$

   D) $5x^3 - 2xc + 10x$

DID YOU KNOW?

You can perform any operation on an equation as long as you do it to both sides of the equation.

Equations

An **equation** includes an equal sign (e.g., $3x + 2xy = 17$) and states that two expressions are equal. Solving an equation means finding the value(s) of the variable that makes the equation true. To do this, isolate the variable on one side of the equation. This can be done by following the same simple steps.

1. Distribute to get rid of parentheses.

2. Use the least common denominator to get rid of fractions.

3. Add/subtract like terms on either side.

4. Add/subtract so that constants appear on only one side of the equation.

5. Multiply/divide to isolate the variable.

$2(2x - 8) = x + 7$	
$4x - 16 = x + 7$	Distribute.
$4x - 16 - x = x + 7 - x$ $3x - 16 = -7$	Subtract x to isolate the variable on one side.
$3x - 16 + 16 = -7 + 16$ $3x = 9$	Add 16 to both sides.
$\frac{3x}{3} = \frac{9}{3}$ $x = 3$	Divide both sides by 3.

PRACTICE QUESTIONS

5. Solve for x: $5(x + 3) - 12 = 43$

A) $x = 3$

B) $x = 8$

C) $x = 10.4$

D) $x = 14$

6. Solve: $-4x + 2 = -34$

A) -9

B) -8

C) 8

D) 9

Graphing Linear Equations on a Coordinate Plane

A **coordinate plane** is a plane containing the x- and y-axes. The x-**axis** is the horizontal line on a graph where $y = 0$. The y-**axis** is the vertical line on a graph where $x = 0$. The x-axis and y-axis intersect to create four **quadrants**. The first quadrant is in the upper right, and other quadrants are labeled counterclockwise using the roman numerals I, II, III, and IV. **Points**, or locations, on the graph are written as **ordered pairs** (x, y), with the point $(0, 0)$ called the **origin**. Points are plotted by counting over x places from the origin horizontally and y places from the origin vertically.

$\longrightarrow$
CONTINUE

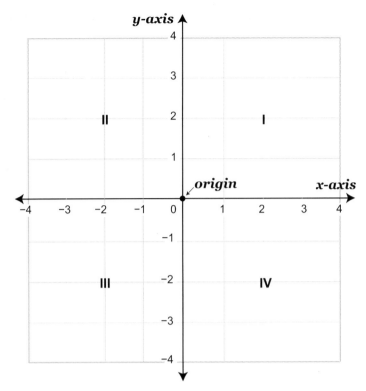

Figure 4.2. The Coordinate Plane

The most common way to write a linear equation is **slope-intercept form**:

$$y = mx + b$$

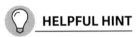

HELPFUL HINT

Use the phrase "begin, move" to remember that b is the y-intercept (where to begin) and m is the slope (how the line moves).

In this equation, m is the slope, and b is the y-intercept. The y-**intercept** is the point where the line crosses the y-axis, or where x equals zero. **Slope** is often described as "rise over run" because it is calculated as the difference in y-values (rise) over the difference in x-values (run).

$$m = \frac{y_2 - y_1}{x_2 - x_1} = \frac{\text{rise}}{\text{run}}$$

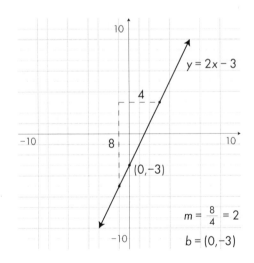

Figure 4.3. Linear Equation

To graph a linear equation, identify the y-intercept and place that point on the y-axis. Then, starting at the y-intercept, use the slope of "rise over run" to go "up and over" and place the next point. The numerator of the slope tells you how many units to go up, the "rise." The denominator of the slope tells you how many units to go to the right, the "run." However, if the slope is negative, you must reverse the process and go down and over to the left before placing the next point. You can repeat the process to plot additional points. These points can then be connected to draw the line. To find the equation of a line, identify the y-intercept, if possible, on the graph and use two easily identifiable points to find the slope.

 DID YOU KNOW?

Two or more **parallel lines** never intersect, and they have the same or equal slopes. **Perpendicular lines** intersect to form right angles. The slopes of two perpendicular lines are negative reciprocals of each other.

PRACTICE QUESTIONS

7. What is the slope of the line whose equation is $6x - 2y - 8 = 0$?

A) -3

B) $-1/3$

C) 3

D) $\frac{3}{4}$

8. In which quadrant is the point $(-5, 2)$ located?

A) I

B) II

C) III

D) IV

Inequalities

Inequalities look like equations, except that instead of having an equal sign, they have one of the following symbols:

- $>$ Greater than: The expression left of the symbol is larger than the expression on the right.

- $<$ Less than: The expression left of the symbol is smaller than the expression on the right.

- $\geq$ Greater than or equal to: The expression left of the symbol is larger than or equal to the expression on the right.

- $\leq$ Less than or equal to: The expression left of the symbol is less than or equal to the expression on the right.

Inequalities are solved like linear and algebraic equations. The only difference is that the symbol must be reversed when both sides of the equation are multiplied or divided by a negative number.

$$10 - 2x > 14$$
$$-2x > 4$$
$$x < -2$$

The solution to an inequality is a *set* of numbers, not a single value. In the example above, the answer $x < -2$ means that all numbers less than -2 make the inequality true.

PRACTICE QUESTION

9. Solve the inequality: $4x + 10 > 58$

   A) $x > 12$

   B) $x < 12$

   C) $x > 19.5$

   D) $x > 11$

Building Equations

Any of the math concepts discussed here can be turned into a word problem that requires you to translate words into a mathematical expression, equation, or inequality. Most of these problems can be solved using these general steps:

- **Step 1**: Read the entire problem and determine what the question is asking for.

- **Step 2**: List all the given data and define the variables.

- **Step 3**: Determine the formula needed or set up equations from the information in the problem.

- **Step 4**: Solve.

- **Step 5**: Check your answer. (Is the amount too large or too small? Are the answers in the correct unit of measure?)

Word problems generally contain key words that can help you determine what math processes may be required in order to solve them. These will help you in Step 3, when you need to build an equation or inequality.

TABLE 4.1. Translating Word Problems	
ENGLISH WORDS AND PHRASES	**MATH TRANSLATION**
is, will be, yields, amounts to, equals	$=$
y is at least (or no less than) x	$y \geq x$
y is at most (or no more than) x	$y \leq x$
in addition to, increased by, added to, perimeter, sum, total, in all	$+$
less, fewer, how much more, difference, decreased	$-$
of, times, area, product	$\times$
distribute, share, per, out of	$\div$
opposite of x	$-x$
ratio of x to y	$\frac{x}{y}$

10. Bob's hospital bill is $1,896. If Bob pays $158 per month, which expression represents his balance after x months?

A) $1896 - 158x$

B) $158x + 1896$

C) $1738x$

D) $158(1896 - x)$

11. The students on the track team are buying new uniforms. T-shirts (t) cost $12, pants ($p$) cost $15, and a pair of shoes (s) costs $45. If the team has a budget of $2,500, write a mathematical sentence that represents how many of each item they can buy.

A) $t + p + s < 2500$

B) $\frac{t}{12} + \frac{p}{15} + \frac{s}{45} > 2500$

C) $12t + 15p + 45s < 2500$

D) $12t + 15p + 45s \geq 2500$

Absolute Value

The **absolute value** of a number is the distance between that number and zero. The absolute value of any number is positive since distance is always positive. The notation for absolute value of a number is two vertical bars:

$$|-27| = 27$$
$$|27| = 27$$

Because the number between the bars can have two values (one positive and one negative), solving equations with absolute values requires writing two equations:

$$|x - 3| = 27$$

Equation 1
$$x - 3 = 27$$
$$x = 30$$

Equation 2
$$x - 3 = -27$$
$$x = -24$$

 HELPFUL HINT

The absolute value of a number is just the positive form of the value within the bars.

→
CONTINUE

PRACTICE QUESTION

12. Solve for r:

$|r - 7| = 135$

A) $\{-128, 128\}$

B) $\{128, -142\}$

C) $\{135, 142\}$

D) $\{-128, 142\}$

Answer Key

1. **D)** Substitute the value -10 for a in the expression and simplify:

$\frac{a^2}{4} - 3a + 4$

$= \frac{(-10)^2}{4} - 3(-10) + 4$

$= \frac{100}{4} + 30 + 4$

$= 25 + 30 + 4 = \mathbf{59}$

2. **A)** Substitute the given terms for a and b:

$2a + 3b$

$= 2(xy) + 3(x^2)$

$= \mathbf{2xy + 3x^2}$

3. **A)** Combine like terms:

$4x - 3y + 12z + 2x - 7y - 10z$

$= (4x + 2x) + (-3y - 7y) + (12z - 10z)$

$= \mathbf{6x - 10y + 2z}$

4. **B)** Distribute the term $5x$ by multiplying by each of the three terms inside the parentheses:

$5x(x^2 - 2c + 10)$

$(5x)(x^2) = 5x^3$

$(5x)(-2c) = -10xc$

$(5x)(10) = 50x$

$5x(x^2 - 2c + 10)$

$= \mathbf{5x^3 - 10xc + 50x}$

5. **B)** Distribute the 5 and combine like terms:

$5(x + 3) - 12 = 43$

$5x + 15 - 12 = 43$

$5x + 3 = 43$

Subtract 3 from both sides:

$5x + 3 - 3 = 43 - 3$

$5x = 40$

Divide both sides by 5:

$\frac{5x}{5} = \frac{40}{5}$

$\mathbf{x = 8}$

6. **D)** Isolate x by subtracting 2 from each side:

$-4x + 2 = -34$

$-4x = -36$

Divide by -4.

$\mathbf{x = 9}$

7. **C)** Write in slope-intercept form (solve for y):

$6x - 2y - 8 = 0$

$-2y = -6x + 8$

$\frac{-2y}{-2} = \frac{-6x}{-2} + \frac{8}{-2}$

$y = 3x - 4$

The slope is the coefficient of x, which is **3**.

8. **B)** Starting at the origin, move 5 units to the left and then up 2 units. The point is located in the top left quadrant, which is **quadrant II**.

9. **A)** Subtract 10 from both sides:

$4x + 10 > 58$

$4x + 10 - 10 > 58 - 10$

$4x > 48$

Divide by 4 to isolate x:

$\frac{4x}{4} > \frac{48}{4}$

$x > 12$

10. **A)** Multiply the monthly payment by the number of months: $158x$.

Subtract from the total bill: **$1896 - 158x$**.

11. **C)** Identify the quantities:

number of shirts $= t$

total cost of shirts $= 12t$

number of pants $= p$

total cost of pants $= 15p$

number of pairs of shoes $= s$

total cost of shoes $= 45s$

The cost of all the items must be less than \$2,500: **$12t + 15p + 45s < 2500$**

12. **D)** Set up two equations to solve for r.

Equation 1

$r - 7 = 135$

$r = \mathbf{142}$

Equation 2

$r - 7 = -135$

$r = \mathbf{-128}$

5 | Geometry

Units of Measurement

The TEAS will test your knowledge of two types of units: the US customary (or American) system and the metric system (or SI units). The **US system** includes many of the units you likely use in day-to-day activities; these include the foot, pound, and cup. The **metric system** is used throughout most of the rest of the world and is the main system used in science and medicine. Common units for the US and metric systems are shown in Table 5.1.

TABLE 5.1. Units

DIMENSION	US CUSTOMARY	METRIC/SI
Length	inch/foot/yard/mile	meter
Mass	ounce/pound/ton	gram
Volume	cup/pint/quart/gallon	liter
Temperature	Fahrenheit	kelvin, Celsius

The metric system uses prefixes to simplify large and small numbers. These prefixes are added to the base units shown in the table. For example, the measurement "1000 meters" can be written using the prefix *kilo–* as "1 kilometer." The most commonly used SI prefixes are given in Table 5.2.

TABLE 5.2. Metric Prefixes

PREFIX	SYMBOL	MULTIPLICATION FACTOR
kilo	k	1,000
hecto	h	100
deca	da	10
base unit	--	--
deci	d	0.1
centi	c	0.01
milli	m	0.001

 DID YOU KNOW?

The abbreviation "SI" in "SI units" stands for *Système international d'unités,* French for "International System of Units."

Conversion factors can be used to convert between units both within a single system and between the US and metric systems. Some questions on the TEAS will require you to know common conversion factors, some of which are given below.

- 1 in = 2.54 cm
- 1 lb = 0.454 kg
- 1 yd = 0.914 m
- 1 cal = 4.19 J
- 1 mi = 1.61 km
- $C = \frac{5}{9}(^{\circ}F - 32)$
- 1 gal = 3.785 L
- $1 \text{ cm}^3 = 1 \text{ mL}$
- 1 oz = 28.35 g
- 1 hr = 3,600 s

To perform unit conversion, start with the initial value and multiply by a conversion factor to reach the final unit. This process is shown in Figure 5.1.

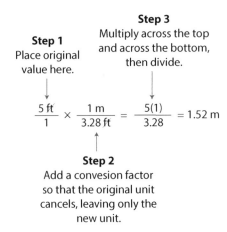

Figure 5.1. Unit Conversion

 HELPFUL HINT

When doing unit conversion, cross out units that appear on the top and bottom. Only the units you want in the answer should be left.

PRACTICE QUESTIONS

1. How many meters are in 4.25 kilometers?

   A) 0.004215 meters

   B) 0.425 meters

   C) 4250 meters

   D) 42,500 meters

2. A ball rolling across a table travels 6 inches per second. How many feet will it travel in 2 minutes?

   A) 1 foot

   B) 30 feet

C) 60 feet

D) 10,800 feet

Lines and Angles

Geometric figures are shapes composed of points, lines, or planes. A **point** is simply a location in space; it does not have any dimensional properties such as length, area, or volume. Points are written as a single capital letter, such as A or Q.

A collection of points that extends infinitely in both directions is a **line**, and one that extends infinitely in only one direction is a **ray**. A section of a line with a beginning and end is a **line segment**. A line segment is described by the beginning and end point, such as AQ. Lines, rays, and line segments are examples of **one-dimensional objects** because they can only be measured in one dimension (length).

Lines, rays, and line segments can intersect to create angles, which are measured in degrees or radians. Angles are classified based on the number of degrees they contain.

- Angles between 0 and 90 degrees are **acute**.
- Angles between 90 and 180 degrees are **obtuse**.
- An angle of exactly 90 degrees is a **right angle**.

Two angles with measurements that add up to 90 degrees are **complementary**, and two angles with measurements that add up to 180 degrees are **supplementary**. Two adjacent (touching) angles are called a **linear pair**, and they are supplementary.

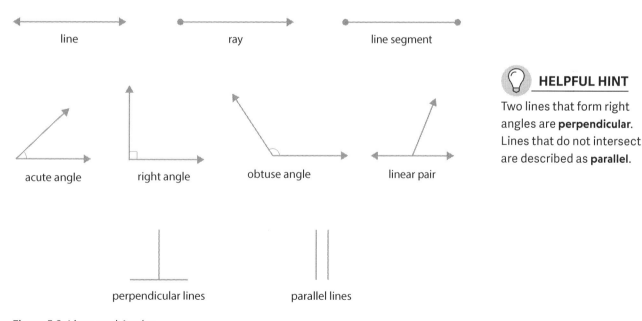

> **HELPFUL HINT**
>
> Two lines that form right angles are **perpendicular**. Lines that do not intersect are described as **parallel**.

Figure 5.2. Lines and Angles

3. A teacher shows her students the angle below and asks them to draw a larger angle.

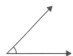

Which of the following student answers is correct?

A)

B)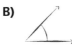

C)

D)

Two-Dimensional Shapes

Two-dimensional objects can be measured in two dimensions (length and width). A **plane** is a two-dimensional object that extends infinitely in both dimensions. **Polygons** are two-dimensional shapes, such as triangles and squares, that have three or more straight sides. **Regular polygons** are polygons with sides that are all the same length.

A **circle** is the set of all the points in a plane that are the same distance from a fixed point (called the **center**). The distance from the center to any point on the circle is the **radius** of the circle. The **diameter** is the largest measurement across a circle. It passes through the circle's center, extending from one side of the circle to the other. The measure of the diameter is twice the measure of the radius. A **sector** is the part of the circle formed by two radii (like a pie slice).

> **HELPFUL HINT**
>
> Because all the points on a circle are equidistant from the center, all the circle's radii have the same length.

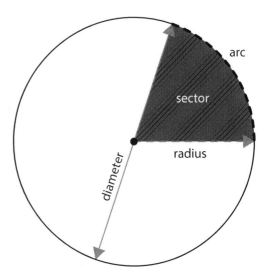

Figure 5.3. Parts of a Circle

Triangles have three sides and three interior angles that always sum to 180°. A **scalene triangle** has no equal sides or angles. An **isosceles triangle** has two equal sides and two equal angles (often called base angles). In an **equilateral triangle**, all three sides are equal, as are all three angles. Moreover, because the sum of the angles of a triangle is always 180°, each angle of an equilateral triangle must be 60°.

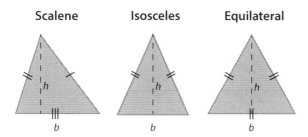

Figure 5.4. Types of Triangles

A **right triangle** has one right angle. The side of the triangle opposite this angle is the **hypotenuse**. The **Pythagorean theorem** gives the relationship between the three sides of a triangle (where c is the hypotenuse):

$$a^2 + b^2 = c^2$$

Quadrilaterals have four sides and four angles.

- In a **rectangle**, each of the four angles measures 90°, and there are two pairs of sides with equal lengths.
- A **square** also has four 90° angles, and all four of its sides are an equal length.
- A **rhombus** has four equal sides and two pairs of equal angles.
- A **trapezoid** has two parallel sides.
- A **parallelogram** has two pairs of parallel, equal sides.

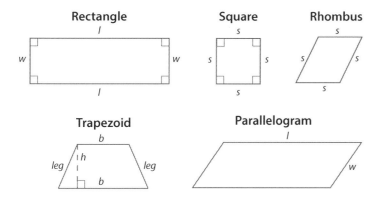

Figure 5.5. Quadrilaterals

The size of the surface of a two-dimensional object is its **area**. The distance around a two-dimensional figure is its **perimeter**, which can be found by adding the lengths of all the sides.

TABLE 5.3. Area and Perimeter of Basic Shapes

SHAPE	AREA	PERIMETER	VARIABLES
Triangle	$A = \frac{1}{2}bh$	$P = s_1 + s_2 + s_3$	b = base
Square	$A = s^2$	$P = 4s$	h = height
			s = side
Rectangle	$A = l \times w$	$P = 2l + 2w$	l = length
Circle	$A = \pi r^2$	$C = 2\pi r$	w = width
			r = radius
			C = circumference
Sector	$A = \frac{x°}{360°}\pi r^2$	$s = \frac{x°}{360°}2\pi r$	$x°$ = angle of sector
			s = arc length
			$\pi \approx 3.14$

The TEAS will include area and perimeter problems with compound shapes. These are complex shapes made by combining more basic shapes. While they might look complicated, they can be solved by simply breaking the compound shape apart and using the formulas given above.

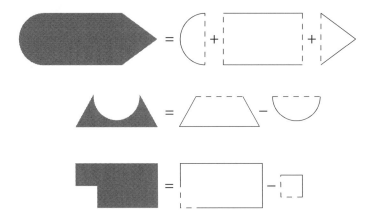

Figure 5.6. Compound Shapes

PRACTICE QUESTIONS

4. Which of the following expressions describes the area of the triangle below?

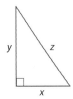

A) $x + y + z$

B) $\frac{xy}{2}$

C) xyz

D) $\frac{xyz}{2}$

5. The figure below shows a circle placed inside a square and tangent to all four sides.

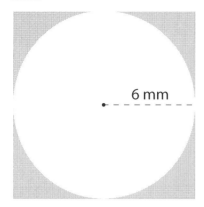

Which of the following is closest to the area of the shaded region?

A) 17.16 mm²

B) 30.96 mm²

C) 106.32 mm²

D) 125.16 mm²

6. Erica is participating in a race in which she'll run 3 miles due north and 4 miles due east. She'll then run back to the starting line. How far will she run during this race?

A) 5 miles

B) 7 miles

C) 12 miles

D) 25 miles

Three-Dimensional Shapes

Three-dimensional objects, like cubes, can be measured in three dimensions (length, width, and height). Three-dimensional objects are also called **solids**, and the shape of a flattened solid is called a **net**.

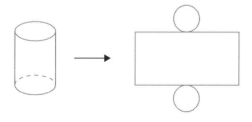

Figure 5.7. Net of a Cylinder

The **surface area** (*SA*) of a three-dimensional object can be figured by adding the areas of all the sides. Surface area is measured in square units (e.g., m² or ft²). **Volume** (*V*) is the amount of space that a three-dimensional object takes up. Volume is measured in cubic units (e.g., ft³ or mm³).

TABLE 5.4. Three-Dimensional Shapes and Formulas

TERM	SHAPE	FORMULA	
Prism		$V = Bh$ $SA = 2lw + 2wh + 2lh$ $d^2 = a^2 + b^2 + c^2$	B = area of base h = height l = length w = width d = longest diagonal
Cube		$V = s^3$ $SA = 6s^2$	s = cube edge
Sphere		$V = \frac{4}{3}\pi r^3$ $SA = 4\pi r^2$	r = radius
Cylinder		$V = Bh = \pi r^2 h$ $SA = 2\pi r^2 + 2\pi rh$	B = area of base h = height r = radius
Cone		$V = \frac{1}{3}\pi r^2 h$ $SA = \pi r^2 + \pi rl$	r = radius h = height l = slant height
Pyramid		$V = \frac{1}{3}Bh$ $SA = B + \frac{1}{2}(p)l$	B = area of base h = height p = perimeter l = slant height

PRACTICE QUESTIONS

7. What is the surface area of a cube with a side length of 5 mm?

A) 75 mm²

B) 100 mm²

C) 125 mm²

D) 150 mm²

8. A rectangular tank with a width of 3 meters and a length of 5 meters is filled with 30 cubic meters of water. What will be the height of the water?

A) 2 meters

B) 18 meters

C) 22 meters

D) 30 meters

Congruency and Similarity

When discussing shapes in geometry, the term **congruent** is used to mean that two shapes have the same shape and size (but not necessarily the same orientation or location). For example, if the lengths of two lines are equal, the two lines themselves are called congruent. Congruence is written using the symbol ≅. On figures, congruent parts are denoted with hash marks (see Figure 5.8).

Shapes that are **similar** have the same shape but not the same size, meaning their corresponding angles are the same but their lengths are not. For two shapes to be similar, the ratio of their corresponding sides must be a constant (called the **scale factor**). Similarity is described using the symbol ~.

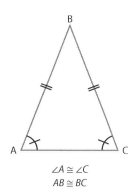

$$\angle A \cong \angle C$$
$$AB \cong BC$$

Figure 5.8. Congruent Parts of a Triangle

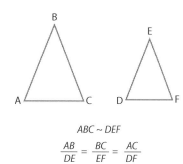

$$ABC \sim DEF$$
$$\frac{AB}{DE} = \frac{BC}{EF} = \frac{AC}{DF}$$

Figure 5.9. Similar Triangles

PRACTICE QUESTION

9. The figure below shows similar triangles *ABC* and *DEF*.

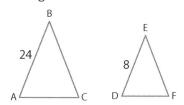

Which of the following statements is true?

A) $DF = \frac{AC}{3}$

B) $DF = AC - 16$

C) $DF = 2AC$

D) $DF = \frac{2}{3}AB$

Answer Key

1. **C)** There are 1000 kilometers in 1 meter, so use the conversion factor $\frac{1,000m}{1km}$.

    $\frac{4.25 \text{ km}}{\blacksquare} \times \frac{1,000m}{1 \text{ km}} = \textbf{4250 meters}$

2. **C)** The rate is given in inches per second, but the question asks for feet per minute. Start by converting the units from inches per second to feet per minute.

    $\frac{6 \text{ in}}{1 \text{ s}} \times \frac{60 \text{ s}}{1 \text{ min}} \times \frac{1 \text{ ft}}{12 \text{ in}} = 30 \text{ ft/min}$

    Multiply the rate by the given amount of time (2 minutes).

    $\frac{2 \text{ min}}{\blacksquare} \times \frac{30 \text{ ft}}{1 \text{ min}} = \textbf{60 feet}$

3. **D)**
    A: This student tried to draw a larger angle by extending the rays farther from the vertex.
    B: This student increased the size of the angle symbol but did not increase the size of the angle.
    C: This student drew a smaller angle.
    D: This student drew a larger angle.

4. **B)** The formula for the area of a triangle is $\frac{1}{2}bh$, where b is the base and h is the height. In this triangle, y is the base and x is the height, so the triangle's area is $\frac{1}{2}xy$, or $\mathbf{\frac{xy}{2}}$.

5. **B)** Find the area of the square:
    $A = s^2 = 12^2 = 144 \text{ mm}^2$
    Find the area of the circle:
    $A = \pi r^2 = \pi(6)^2 = 36\pi \text{ mm}^2$
    Subtract the area of the circle from the square (use 3.14 for π):
    $144 - 36\pi \approx \textbf{30.96 mm}^2$

6. **C)** One leg of her route (the triangle) is missing, but you can find its length using the Pythagorean theorem:
    $a^2 + b^2 = c^2$
    $3^2 + 4^2 = c^2$
    $25 = c^2$
    $c = 5$
    Adding all three sides gives the length of the whole race:
    $3 + 4 + 5 = \textbf{12 miles}$

7. **D)** A cube has six faces, each of which is a square.
    Find the area of each side using the formula for the area of a square:
    $A = s^2 = 5^2 = 25 \text{ mm}^2$
    Multiply the area by 6 (because the cube has six faces):
    $SA = 25(6) = \textbf{150 mm}^2$

8. **A)** Use the formula for the volume of a rectangular solid to solve for the height (h):

$V = wlh$

$30 \text{ m}^3 = (3 \text{ m})(5 \text{ m})(h)$

$h = \textbf{2 meters}$

9. **A)** Use the given lengths to find the scale ratio for the two triangles:

$\frac{AB}{DE} = \frac{24}{8} = 3$

The ratio of DF to AC will also be equal to 3 because they are corresponding parts of the two triangles:

$\frac{AC}{DF} = 3$

Solve for DF:

$DF = \frac{AC}{3}$

6 | Statistics

Measures of Central Tendency

Measures of central tendency help identify the center, or most typical, value within a data set. There are three such central tendencies that describe the "center" of the data in different ways. The **mean** (μ) is the arithmetic average and is found by dividing the sum of all measurements by the number of measurements.

$$\mu = \frac{x_1 + x_2 + \dots x_N}{N}$$

Find the mean of the following data set: {75, 62, 78, 92, 83, 90}

$$\frac{75 + 62 + 78 + 92 + 83 + 90}{6} = \frac{480}{6} = 80$$

The **median** divides a set into two equal halves. To calculate the median, place the data set in ascending order. The median is the measurement right in the middle of an odd set of measurements or the average of the two middle numbers in an even data set.

Find the median of the following data set: {2, 15, 16, 8, 21, 13, 4}

Place the data in ascending order: {2, 4, 8, <u>13</u>, 15, 16, 21}

The median is the value in the middle: 13

Find the median of the following data set: {75, 62, 78, 92, 83, 91}

Place the data in ascending order: {62, 75, <u>78, 83</u>, 91, 92}

Find the average of the two middle values: $\frac{78 + 83}{2} = 80.5$

Outliers are values in a data set that are much larger or smaller than the other values in the set. Outliers can skew the mean, making it higher or lower than most of the values. The median is not affected by outliers, so it is a better measure of central tendency when outliers are present.

For the set {3, 5, 10, 12, 65}:

$$\text{mean} = \frac{3 + 5 + 10 + 12 + 65}{5} = 19$$

 HELPFUL HINT

Adding a constant to each value in a data set will change both the mean and the median by that value. Multiplying each value in a set by a constant will also change the mean and the median by the same value.

$$\text{median} = 10$$

The outlier (65) drags the mean much higher than the median.

The **mode** is simply the measurement that occurs most often. There can be one, several, or no modes in a data set.

PRACTICE QUESTIONS

1. A student has an average of 81 on four equally weighted tests she has taken in her statistics class. What grade must she receive on her fifth test if she needs an average score of 83?

   A) 81

   B) 83

   C) 89

   D) 91

2. What is the median of the following set: {24, 27, 18, 19}?

   A) 19

   B) 21.5

   C) 24

   D) 25.5

Measures of Dispersion

The values in a data set can be very close together (close to the mean) or very spread out. This is called the **spread** or **dispersion** of the data. There are a few **measures of dispersion** that quantify the spread within a data set. **Range** is the difference between the largest and smallest data points in a set:

$$R = \text{largest data point} - \text{smallest data point}$$

Notice range depends on only two data points, the two extremes. Sometimes these data points are outliers; regardless, for a large data set, relying on only two data points is not an exact tool. To better understand the data set, calculate **quartiles**, which divide data sets into four equally sized groups. To calculate quartiles:

1. Arrange the data in ascending order.

2. Find the set's median (also called quartile 2 or Q2).

3. Find the median of the lower half of the data, called quartile 1 (Q1).

4. Find the median of the upper half of the data, called quartile 3 (Q3).

The **interquartile range (IQR)** provides a more reliable range that is not as affected by extremes. IQR is the difference between the third quartile data point and the first quartile data point:

$$IQR = Q_3 - Q_1$$

3. The table below shows the number of customers that came into a restaurant each day of the week.

DAY of the Week	NUMBER of Customers
Monday	72
Tuesday	89
Wednesday	125
Thursday	212
Friday	350
Saturday	418
Sunday	262

What is the range of the data set?

A) 72

B) 218

C) 281

D) 346

Data Presentation

Bar graphs present the numbers of an item that exist in different categories. The categories are shown on one axis, and the number of items is shown on the other axis. Bar graphs are usually used to compare amounts easily.

Histograms similarly use bars to compare data, but the independent variable is a continuous variable that has been "binned" or divided into categories. For example, the time of day can be broken down into 8:00 a.m. to 12:00 p.m., 12:00 p.m. to 4:00 p.m., and so on. Usually (but not always), a gap is included between the bars of a bar graph, but not a histogram.

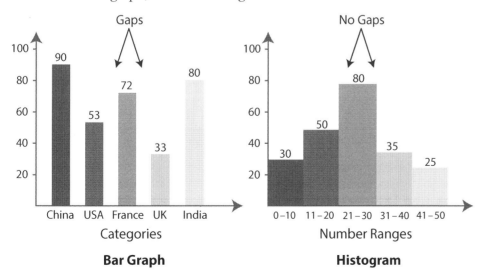

Figure 6.1. Bar Graph versus Histogram

Scatter plots show the relationship between two sets of data by plotting the data as ordered pairs (x, y). One variable is plotted along the horizontal axis, and the second variable is plotted along the vertical axis.

The data in a scatter plot may show a **linear relationship** between the data sets. There is a **positive correlation** (expressed as a positive slope) if increasing one variable corresponds to an increase in the other variable. A **negative correlation** (expressed as a negative slope) occurs when an increase in one variable corresponds to a decrease in the other. If the scatter plot shows no discernible pattern, then there is no correlation (a zero, mixed, or indiscernible slope).

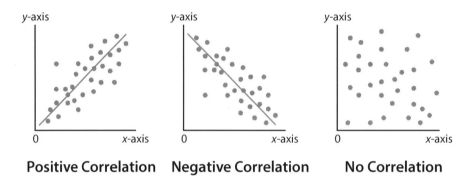

Positive Correlation   Negative Correlation   No Correlation

Figure 6.2. Scatter Plots and Correlation

Correlation is a mathematical term that describes two variables that are statistically related (meaning one variable can be used to predict the other). **Causation** means that one variable directly influences another through a known mechanism. Correlation is not the same as causation: knowing two variables are statistically related does not mean one is directly influencing the other.

Line graphs are used to display a relationship between two continuous variables, such as change over time. Line graphs are constructed by graphing each point and connecting each point to the next consecutive point by a line.

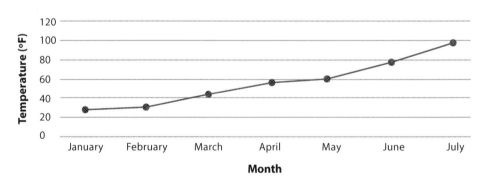

Figure 6.3. Line Graph

Pie charts show parts of a whole and are often used with percentages. Together, all the slices of the pie add up to the total number of items, or 100%.

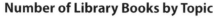

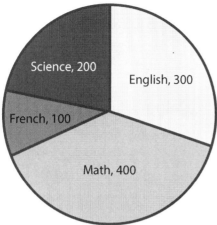

Figure 6.4. Pie Chart

Stem-and-leaf plots are ways of organizing large amounts of data by grouping it into rows. All data points are broken into two parts: a stem and a leaf. For instance, the number 512 might be broken into a stem of 5 and a leaf of 12. All data in the 500 range would appear in the same row (this group of data is a class). The advantage of this display is that it shows general density and shape of the data in a compact display, yet all original data points are preserved and available. It is also easy to find medians and quartiles from this display.

STEM	LEAF
0	5
1	6, 7
2	8, 3, 6
3	4, 5, 9, 5, 5, 8, 5
4	7, 7, 7, 8
5	5, 4
6	0

Figure 6.5. Stem and Leaf Plot

CONTINUE

PRACTICE QUESTIONS

4. The graph below shows rainfall in inches per month.

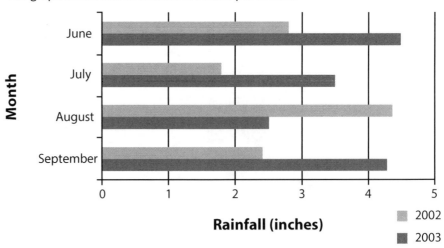

Which month had the highest total rainfall in 2002?

A) June

B) July

C) August

D) September

5. The graph below shows the average high temperature in Houston, Texas, for each month.

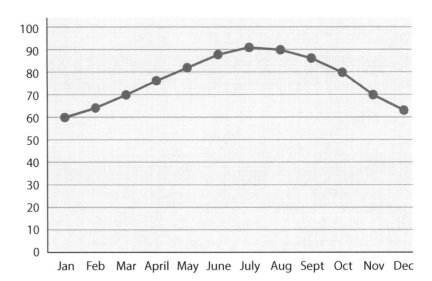

Which of the following is closest to the range for this data set?

A) 15

B) 30

C) 60

D) 90

6. The stem-and-leaf plot below shows students' scores on a recent math test.

9	9, 8, 8, 5, 2, 1
8	8, 8, 8, 4, 2
7	9, 8, 6, 2
6	7, 7, 3
5	5

9|9 = 99

What was the median student score on the test?

A) 82

B) 84

C) 88

D) 91

Data Distribution

Trends in a data set can also be seen by graphing the data as a dot plot or bar graph. The shape of the graph can then be used to identify trends in data distribution. A **symmetric distribution** is equally weighted across the data set. A **skewed distribution** is weighted more heavily toward the right or the left. Right skew describes a data set with fewer points on the right; left skew describes a data set with fewer points on the left. In a **uniform** data set, the points are distributed evenly along the graph.

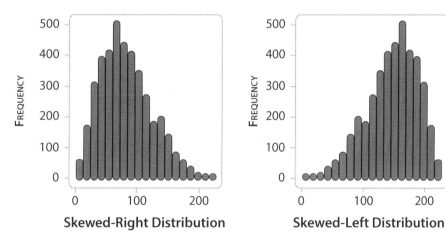

Figure 6.6. Skewed Distribution

A symmetric or skewed distribution may have **peaks,** or sets of data points that appear more frequently. A **unimodal** distribution has one peak while a **bimodal** distribution has two peaks. A **normal** (or bell-shaped) distribution is a special symmetric, unimodal graph with a specific distribution of data points.

CONTINUE

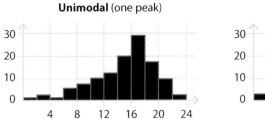

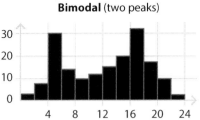

Figure 6.7. Unimodal and Bimodal Distribution

PRACTICE QUESTION

7. Which of the following best describes the distribution of the following graph?

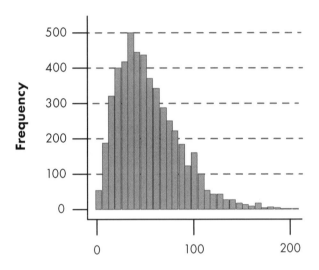

A) skewed left

B) skewed right

C) bimodal

D) uniform

Answer Key

1. **D)** If she has an average of 81 on four tests, then the sum of her scores on the first four tests will be 4×81.

$$\mu = \frac{x_1 + x_2 + \ldots x_N}{N}$$

$$81 = \frac{x_1 + x_2 + x_3 + x_4}{4}$$

$$x_1 + x_2 + x_3 + x_4 = 4(81)$$

Set up a new equation to find the score she needs on her fifth test (x_5) to have an average of 83.

$$\frac{4(81) + x}{5} = 83$$

$$324 + x = 415$$

$$x = 91$$

The student must score a **91** on the last test to have a mean score of 83.

2. **B)** Place the terms in ascending order. Because there are an even number of terms, the median will be the average of the middle 2 terms:

18, 19, 24, 27

$$\text{median} = \frac{19 + 24}{2} = \mathbf{21.5}$$

3. **D)** Subtract the lowest value from the highest value.

$418 - 72 = \mathbf{346}$

4. **C)** The key shows that the light-gray top bar represents 2002. The longest bar for 2002 is in **August**, corresponding to approximately 4.3 inches of rain.

5. **B)** The highest temperature is around 90°F, and the lowest temperature is around 60°F. Subtract to find the range:

$90 - 60 = \mathbf{30}$

6. **B)** Count the number of scores: there are nineteen total values in the set. Count from the top or bottom to find the middle (tenth) value:

9	9, 8, 8, 5, 2, 1
8	8, 8, 8, **4**, 2
7	9, 8, 6, 2
6	7, 7, 3
5	5

9|9 = 99

7. **B)** The graph is skewed right because there are fewer data points on the right half and more on the left half.

PART

3 | Science

The ATI TEAS Science test includes questions on a range of topics from the life and physical sciences. The distribution of the questions is shown below.

- human anatomy and physiology: eighteen questions
- biology: nine questions
- chemistry: eight questions
- scientific reasoning: nine questions

This might seem overwhelming, but don't worry. The ATI TEAS focuses on only a few important concepts from these fields, making it easier to prepare. These topics include:

- macromolecules (e.g., carbohydrates and proteins)
- genetics
- atomic structure
- physical properties and states of matter
- chemical reactions and bonding

7 Human Anatomy and Physiology

The Biological Hierarchy

The biological hierarchy is a systematic breakdown of the structures of the human body organized from smallest to largest (or largest to smallest). The human body is made up of small units called cells. A **cell** is a microscopic, self-replicating, structural, and functional unit of the body that performs many different jobs. The cell is made up of many smaller units that are sometimes considered to be part of the biological hierarchy, including cytoplasm, organelles, nuclei, and a membrane that separates the cell contents from their surroundings.

Tissues compose the next-largest group of structures in the body. They are a collection of cells that all perform a similar function. The human body has four basic types of tissue:

- **Connective tissues**—which include bones, ligaments, and cartilage—support, separate, or connect the body's various organs and tissues.

- **Epithelial tissues** are thin layers of cells that line blood vessels, body cavities, and some organs.

- **Muscular tissues** contain contractile units that pull on connective tissues to create movement.

- **Nervous tissues** make up the peripheral nervous systems that transmit impulses throughout the body.

After tissues, **organs** are the next-largest structure in the biological hierarchy. Organs are a collection of tissues within the body that share a similar function. For example, the esophagus is an organ whose primary function is carrying food and liquids from the mouth to the stomach.

Organ systems, a group of organs that work together to perform a similar function, rank above organs as the next-largest structure on the biological hierarchy. The esophagus is part of the digestive organ system, which is the entire group of organs in the body that processes food from start to finish.

Finally, an **organism** is the total collection of all the parts of the biological hierarchy working together to form a living being; it is the largest structure in the biological hierarchy.

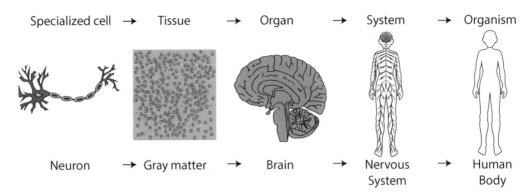

Figure 7.1. Biological Hierarchy

PRACTICE QUESTION

1. The meninges are membranes that surround and protect the brain and spinal cord. What type of tissue would the meninges be classified as?

   A) connective tissues

   B) epithelial tissues

   C) muscular tissues

   D) nervous tissues

✓ **CHECK YOUR UNDERSTANDING**

How would you use anatomical terms to describe the relative positions of the heart and lungs?

Directional Terminology

When discussing anatomy and physiology, specific terms are used to refer to directions. Directional terms include the following:

- **inferior**: away from the head
- **superior**: closer to the head
- **anterior**: toward the front
- **posterior**: toward the back
- **ventral**: toward the front
- **dorsal**: toward the back
- **medial**: toward the midline of the body
- **lateral**: farther from the midline of the body
- **proximal**: closer to the trunk
- **distal**: away from the trunk

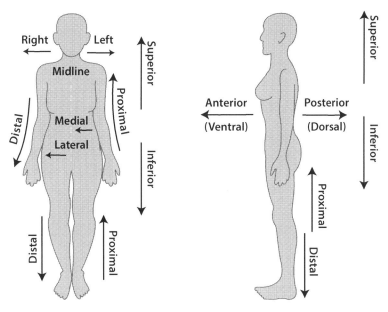

Figure 7.2. Directional Terminology

PRACTICE QUESTION

2.   Where is the wrist located relative to the elbow?

   A) distal

   B) proximal

   C) anterior

   D) posterior

Body Cavities and Planes

The internal structure of the human body is organized into compartments called **cavities**, which are separated by membranes. There are two main cavities in the human body: the **dorsal cavity** and the **ventral cavity** (both named for their relative positions).

The dorsal cavity is further divided into the **cranial cavity**, which holds the brain, and the **spinal cavity**, which surrounds the spine. The two sections of the dorsal cavity are continuous.

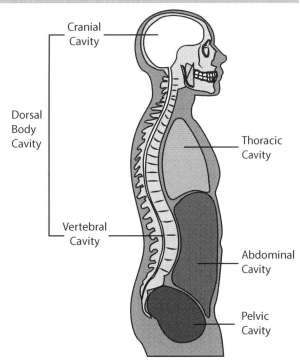

Figure 7.3. Body Cavities

Both sections are lined by the **meninges,** a three-layered membrane that protects the brain and spinal cord.

The ventral cavity houses most of the body's organs. It can be further divided into smaller cavities. The **thoracic cavity** holds the heart and lungs, the **abdominal cavity** holds the digestive organs and kidneys, and the **pelvic cavity** holds the bladder and reproductive organs. Both the abdominal and pelvic cavities are enclosed by a membrane called the **peritoneum.**

The human body is divided by three imaginary planes.

- The **transverse plane** divides the body into a top and bottom half.

- The **frontal** (or coronal) **plane** divides the body into a front and back half.

- The **sagittal plane** divides the body into a right and left half.

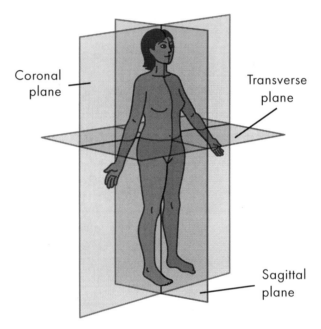

Figure 7.4. Planes of the Human Body

PRACTICE QUESTION

3. Which body cavity holds the appendix?

    A) dorsal

    B) thoracic

    C) abdominal

    D) pelvic

The Cardiovascular System

Structure and Function of the Cardiovascular System

The **cardiovascular system** circulates **blood**, which carries nutrients, wastes, hormones, and other important substances dissolved or suspended in liquid plasma. Two of the most important components of blood are **white blood cells**, which fight infections, and **red blood cells** (RBCs), which transport oxygen. Red blood cells contain **hemoglobin**, a large molecule that includes iron atoms, which binds to oxygen.

Blood is circulated by a muscular organ called the **heart**. The human heart has four chambers, the right and left **atria** and the right and left **ventricles**, as shown in Figure 7.5. Each chamber is isolated by valves that prevent the backflow of blood once it has passed through. The **tricuspid** and **mitral valves** separate atria from ventricles, and the **pulmonary** and **aortic valves** regulate the movement of blood out of the heart into the arteries. The pumping action of the heart is regulated primarily by two neurological **nodes**, the **sinoatrial** and the **atrioventricular** nodes, whose electrical activity sets the rhythm of the heart.

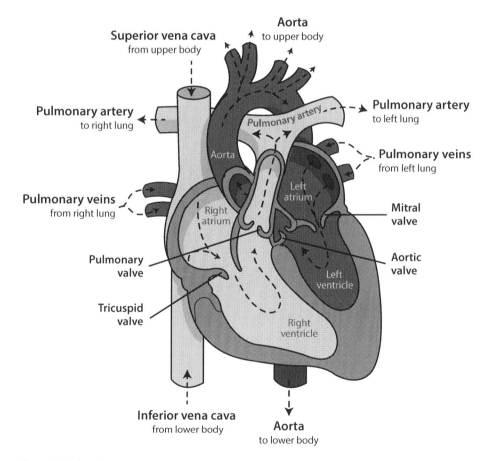

Figure 7.5. The Heart

The heart includes several layers of tissue:

- **pericardium**: the outermost protective layer of the heart that contains a lubricative liquid

- **epicardium**: the deepest layer of the pericardium that envelops the heart muscle

- **myocardium**: the heart muscle

- **endocardium**: the innermost, smooth layer of the heart walls

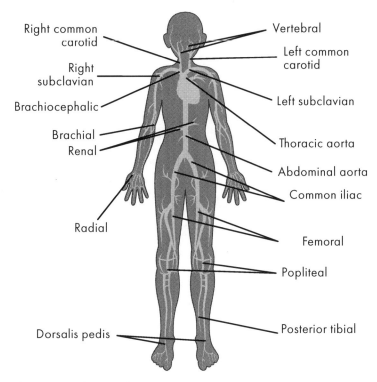

Figure 7.6. Major Arteries

Blood leaves the heart and travels throughout the body in blood vessels, which decrease in diameter as they move away from the heart and toward the tissues and organs. Blood exits the heart through **arteries**, which become **arterioles** and then **capillaries**, the smallest branch of the circulatory system in which gas exchange from

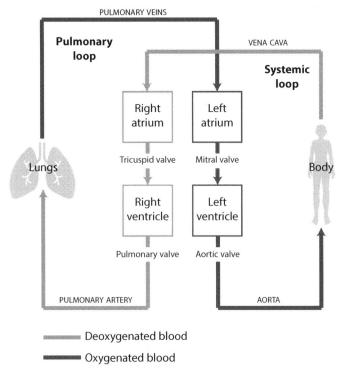

Figure 7.7. Path of Blood Flow Through the Cardiovascular System

blood to tissues occurs. Deoxygenated blood travels back to the heart through **veins**.

The circulatory system includes two closed loops. In the **pulmonary loop**, deoxygenated blood leaves the heart and travels to the lungs, where it loses carbon dioxide and becomes rich in oxygen. The oxygenated blood then returns to the heart, which pumps it through the systemic loop. The **systemic loop** delivers oxygen to the rest of the body and returns deoxygenated blood to the heart.

The Lymphatic System

The **lymphatic system** operates alongside the circulatory system to move fluids and other substances through a system of **lymphatic vessels**. It is particularly important for immune system functioning because it circulates white blood cells. It also removes waste products and balances fluid levels by removing excess interstitial fluid (the fluid between cells).

Lymph, the fluid carried through the lymphatic system, passes through lymph nodes. These nodes filter waste from the lymph and are also home to large numbers of white blood cells. After it has been filtered, lymph is returned to the cardiovascular system through the subclavian vein.

Pathologies of the Cardiovascular System

Hypertension is increased blood pressure, usually above 140/80 mm Hg. Hypertension usually has no symptoms, but it has been linked to heart disease and stroke. **Hypotension** is decreased blood pressure, usually below 90/60 mm Hg.

Ischemia is reduced or restricted blood flow to tissues, and **infarction** is the death of tissue caused by restricted blood flow and the subsequent lack of oxygen. Causes of ischemia include:

- occlusion of blood vessels by an **embolus** (a mass made of fat, bacteria, or other materials) or a **thrombus** (blood clot; also called a thromboembolism)
- narrowed blood vessel (e.g., aneurysm or atherosclerosis)
- trauma

A **myocardial infarction** (MI; also called a heart attack) is an occlusion of the coronary arteries, which supply blood to the heart. The resulting death of cardiac tissue may lead to dysrhythmias, reduced cardiac output, or cardiac arrest. Patients with MI require immediate medical intervention to restore blood flow to the coronary arteries.

Atherosclerosis is a progressive condition in which **plaque** (composed of fat, white blood cells, and other waste) builds up in the arteries. The presence of advanced atherosclerosis places patients at a high risk for several cardiovascular conditions, including blocked or narrowed blood vessels.

Dysrhythmias are abnormal heart rhythms.

- **Bradycardia** is a heart rate < 60 bpm, and **tachycardia** is a heart rate > 100 bpm.

- **Ventricular fibrillation (V-fib)** and **ventricular tachycardia (V-tach)** are dangerous types of tachycardia that can be corrected with shocks from an automatic external defibrillator (AED).

- **Asystole**, also called a "flat line," occurs when there is no electrical or mechanical activity within the heart. It is a non-shockable rhythm with a poor survival rate.

Heart failure occurs when either one or both of the ventricles in the heart cannot efficiently pump blood. Because the heart is unable to pump effectively, blood and fluid back up into the lungs (causing pulmonary congestion), or the fluid builds up peripherally (causing edema of the lower extremities). Heart failure is most commonly categorized into left-sided heart failure or right-sided heart failure, although both sides of the heart can fail at the same time.

Hemophilia is a recessive X-chromosome–linked bleeding disorder characterized by the lack of coagulation factors. **Sickle cell disease** is an inherited form of hemolytic anemia that causes deformities in the shape of the RBCs.

PRACTICE QUESTIONS

4. Which of the following layers of the wall of the heart contains cardiac muscles?

   A) myocardium

   B) epicardium

   C) endocardium

   D) pericardium

5. The blood from the right ventricle goes to

   A) the left atria.

   B) the vena cava.

   C) the aorta.

   D) the lungs.

6. The blood vessels that carry the blood from the heart are called

   A) veins.

   B) venules.

   C) capillaries.

   D) arteries.

The Respiratory System

Structure and Function of the Respiratory System

The **respiratory system** is responsible for the exchange of gases between the human body and the environment. **Oxygen** is brought into the body for use in glucose metabolism, and the **carbon dioxide** created by glucose metabolism is expelled. Gas exchange takes place in the **lungs**. Humans have two lungs, a right

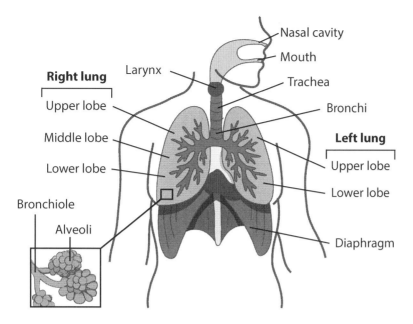

Figure 7.8. The Respiratory System

and a left, and the right lung is slightly larger than the left. The right lung has three **lobes**, and the left has two. The lungs are surrounded by a thick membrane called the **pleura**.

Respiration begins with **pulmonary ventilation**, or breathing. The first stage of breathing is **inhalation**. During this process, the thoracic cavity expands and the diaphragm muscle contracts, which decreases the pressure in the lungs, pulling in air from the atmosphere. Air is drawn in through the nose and mouth, then into the throat, where cilia and mucus filter out particles before the air enters the **trachea**. During inspiration, the **epiglottis** covers the esophagus so that air does not enter the digestive track.

Once it passes through the trachea, the air passes through either the left or right **bronchi**, which are divisions of the trachea that direct air into the left or right lung. These bronchi are further divided into smaller **bronchioles**, which branch throughout the lungs and become increasingly small.

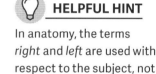

HELPFUL HINT

In anatomy, the terms *right* and *left* are used with respect to the subject, not the observer.

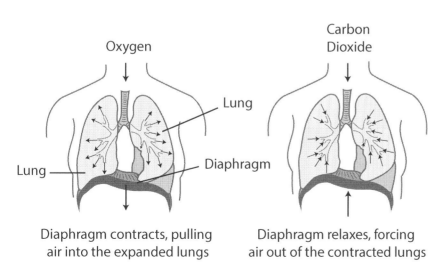

Diaphragm contracts, pulling air into the expanded lungs

Diaphragm relaxes, forcing air out of the contracted lungs

Figure 7.9. The Breathing Process

Eventually, air enters the **alveoli**—tiny air sacs located at the ends of the smallest bronchioles. The alveoli have very thin membranes, only one cell thick, and are the location of gas exchange with the blood: oxygen diffuses into the blood while carbon dioxide is diffused out.

Carbon dioxide is then expelled from the lungs during **exhalation**, the second stage of breathing. During exhalation, the diaphragm relaxes and the thoracic cavity contracts, causing air to leave the body, as the lung pressure is now greater than the atmospheric pressure.

Pathologies of the Respiratory System

Lung diseases that result in the continual restriction of airflow are known as **chronic obstructive pulmonary disease (COPD)**. These include **emphysema**, which is the destruction of lung tissues, and **asthma**, in which the airways are compromised due to a dysfunctional immune response. The main causes of COPD are smoking and air pollution, and genetic factors can also influence the severity of the disease.

A **pulmonary embolism** is a blood clot (usually originating in the legs) that travels to the lungs, causing chest pain, shortness of breath, and low blood oxygen levels.

The respiratory system is also prone to **respiratory tract infections**, with upper respiratory tract infections affecting air inputs in the nose and throat, and lower respiratory tract infections affecting the lungs and their immediate pulmonary inputs. Viral infections of the respiratory system include **influenza** and the **common cold**; bacterial infections include **tuberculosis** and **pertussis** (whooping cough). **Pneumonia**, the inflammation of the lungs that affects alveoli, can be caused by bacteria, viruses, fungi, or parasites. It is often seen in people whose respiratory system has been weakened by other conditions.

Lung cancer is the second-most common type of cancer diagnosed in the United States. (Breast cancer is the most common.) Symptoms of lung cancer include cough, chest pain, and wheezing. Lung cancer is most often caused by smoking, but it can develop in nonsmokers as well.

PRACTICE QUESTIONS

7. During respiration, the epiglottis prevents air from entering which of the following organs?

   A) bronchi

   B) pharynx

   C) larynx

   D) esophagus

8. Which of the following structures are small air sacs that function as the site of gas exchange in the lungs?

   A) capillaries

   B) bronchi

C) alveoli

D) cilia

9. Which of the following conditions is caused by an immune response?

A) COPD

B) influenza

C) asthma

D) emphysema

The Nervous System

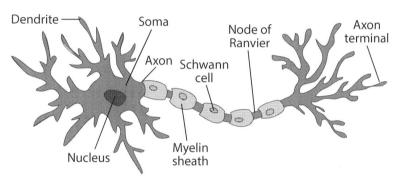

Figure 7.10. The Structure of a Neuron

Structure and Function of the Nervous System

The **nervous system** coordinates the processes and actions of the human body. **Nerve cells**, or **neurons**, communicate through electrical impulses and allow the body to process and respond to stimuli. Neurons have a nucleus and transmit electrical impulses through their axons and dendrites. The **axon** is the stemlike structure, often covered in a fatty insulating substance called **myelin**, that carries information to other neurons throughout the body. Myelin is produced by **Schwann cells**, which also play an important role in nerve regeneration. **Dendrites** receive information from other neurons.

The nervous system is broken down into two parts: the **central nervous system (CNS)** and the **peripheral nervous system (PNS)**. The CNS is made up of the brain and spinal cord. The

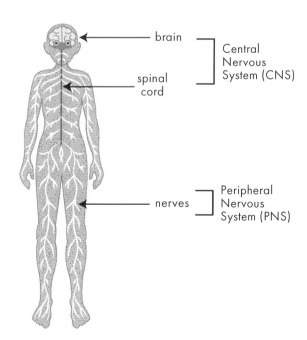

Figure 7.11. The Nervous System

brain acts as the control center for the body and is responsible for nearly all the body's processes and actions. The spinal cord relays information between the brain and the peripheral nervous system; it also coordinates many reflexes. The spinal cord is protected by the vertebral column, a structure of bones that enclose the delicate nervous tissue. The PNS is the collection of nerves that connect the central nervous system to the rest of the body.

The functions of the nervous system are broken down into the autonomic nervous system and the somatic nervous system. The **autonomic nervous system** controls involuntary actions that occur in the body, such as respiration, heartbeat, digestive processes, and more. The **somatic nervous system** is responsible for the body's ability to control skeletal muscles and voluntary movement as well as the involuntary reflexes associated with skeletal muscles.

The autonomic nervous system is further broken down into the sympathetic nervous system and the parasympathetic nervous system. The **sympathetic nervous system** is responsible for the body's reaction to stress and induces a "fight-or-flight" response to stimuli. For instance, if an individual is frightened, the sympathetic nervous system causes an increase in the person's heart rate and blood pressure to prepare them to either fight or flee.

In contrast, the **parasympathetic nervous system** is stimulated by the body's need for rest or recovery. The parasympathetic nervous system responds by decreasing heart rate, blood pressure, and muscular activation when a person is getting ready for activities such as sleeping or digesting food. For example, the body activates the parasympathetic nervous system after eating a large meal, which is why people then feel sluggish.

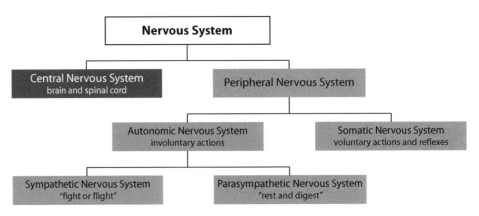

DID YOU KNOW?

The fight-or-flight reaction includes accelerated breathing and heart rate, dilation of blood vessels in muscles, release of energy molecules for use by muscles, relaxation of the bladder, and slowed or stopped movement in the upper digestive tract.

Pathologies of the Nervous System

A **stroke**, or **cardiovascular accident (CVA)**, occurs when blood flow to brain tissue is disrupted. An **ischemic stroke** is the result of a blockage (embolus) in the vasculature of the brain. A **hemorrhagic stroke** is bleeding in the brain, often caused by a ruptured aneurysm.

Figure 7.12. Divisions of the Nervous System

The nervous system can be affected by a number of degenerative diseases that result from the gradual breakdown of nervous tissue. These include:

- **Parkinson's disease**: caused by cell death in the basal ganglia; characterized by gradual loss of motor function

- **multiple sclerosis (MS)**: caused by damage to the myelin sheath; characterized by muscle spasms and weakness, numbness, loss of coordination, and blindness

- **amyotrophic lateral sclerosis (ALS)**: caused by the death of neurons that control voluntary muscle movement; characterized by muscle stiffness, twitches, and weakness

- **Alzheimer's disease**: caused by damaged neurons in the cerebral cortex; characterized by memory loss, confusion, mood swings, and problems with language

The nervous system is also susceptible to infections, some of which can be life threatening. **Meningitis** is inflammation of the meninges, the protective membrane that surrounds the brain and spinal cord, and **encephalitis** is inflammation of the brain. Both conditions can be caused by viral or bacterial pathogens.

Epileptic seizures are brief episodes caused by disturbed or overactive nerve cell activity in the brain. Seizures range widely in severity and may include confusion, convulsions, and loss of consciousness. They have many causes, including tumors, infections, head injuries, and medications.

PRACTICE QUESTIONS

10. Which of the following parts of a neuron is responsible for carrying information away from the cell?

    A) soma

    B) axon

    C) dendrite

    D) myelin

11. Which part of the nervous system controls only voluntary action?

    A) the peripheral nervous system

    B) the somatic nervous system

    C) the sympathetic nervous system

    D) the parasympathetic nervous system

12. What substance does a Schwann cell secrete that increases the speed of signals traveling to and from neurons?

    A) myelin

    B) cerebrospinal fluid

    C) corpus callosum

    D) collagen

Structure and Function of the Skeletal System

The skeletal system is made up of over 200 different **bones**, a stiff connective tissue in the human body with many functions, including:

- protecting internal organs

- synthesizing blood cells

- storing necessary minerals, particularly calcium

- providing the muscular system with leverage to create movement

Bones are covered with a thin layer of vascular connective tissue called the **periosteum**, which serves as a point of muscle attachment, supplies blood to the bone, and contains nerve endings. **Osseous tissue** is the primary tissue that makes up bone. There are two types of osseous tissue: cortical (compact) bone and cancellous (spongy) bone. **Cortical bone** is the dense, solid material that surrounds the bone and gives it hardness and strength. It is usually concentrated in the middle part of the bone.

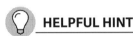

HELPFUL HINT

Osteoclasts are a type of bone cell responsible for breaking down bone tissue. They are located on the surface of bones and help balance the body's calcium levels by degrading bone to release stored calcium.

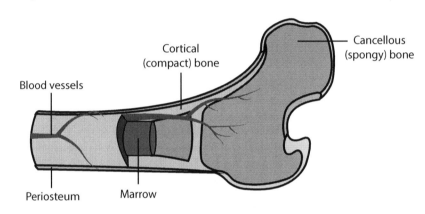

Figure 7.13. Structure of Bone

Cancellous bone is less dense, more porous, and softer. It is located at the ends of long bones, where it does not bear a structural load. Instead, it is a site of the bone's blood production and metabolic activity, as it stores both blood vessels and **bone marrow**. **Red bone marrow** houses **stem cells**, which are made into red blood cells, platelets, and white blood cells (a process called hematopoiesis). **Yellow bone marrow** is composed mostly of fat tissue and can be converted to red bone marrow in response to extreme blood loss in the body.

TABLE 7.1. Types of Bones

NAME	SHAPE	EXAMPLE
Long bones	longer than they are wide	femur, humerus
Short bones	wider than they are long	clavicle, carpals
Flat bones	wide and flat	skull, pelvis
Irregular bones	irregularly shaped	vertebrae, jaw

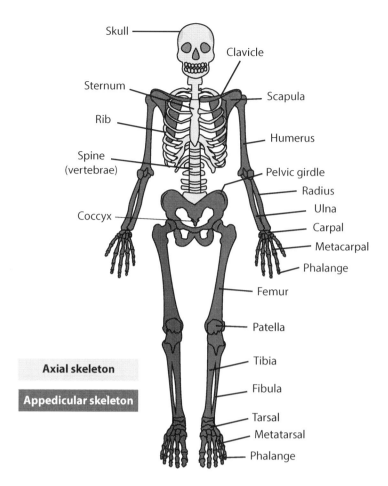

Skull

Clavicle

Sternum

Scapula

Rib

Humerus

Spine (vertebrae)

Pelvic girdle

Radius

Ulna

Coccyx

Carpal

Metacarpal

Phalange

Femur

Patella

Tibia

Fibula

Axial skeleton

Appedicular skeleton

Tarsal

Metatarsal

Phalange

Figure 7.14. The Axial and Appendicular Skeletons

The hundreds of bones in the body make up the human **skeleton**. The **axial skeleton** contains eighty bones and has three major subdivisions: the **skull**, which contains the cranium and facial bones; the **thorax**, which includes the sternum and twelve pairs of ribs; and the **vertebral column**, which contains the body's thirty-three vertebrae. These eighty bones function together to support and protect many of the body's vital organs, including the brain, lungs, heart, and spinal cord. The **appendicular skeleton**'s 126 bones make up the body's appendages. The main function of the appendicular skeleton is locomotion.

Various connective tissues join the parts of the skeleton to other systems, as shown in the table below.

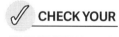 **CHECK YOUR UNDERSTANDING**

How might diet affect the body's ability to rebuild bone after a fracture?

TABLE 7.2. Connective Tissue in the Skeletal System	
TISSUE	**FUNCTION**
Ligament	Joins bone to bone.
Tendon	Joins bones to muscles.
Cartilage	Cushions bones in joints. Provides structural integrity for many body parts (e.g., the ears and nose) and maintains open pathways (e.g., the trachea and bronchi).

Joints

The point at which a bone is attached to another bone is called a joint. There are three basic types of joints:

- **Fibrous joints** connect bones that do not move.
- **Cartilaginous joints** connect bones with cartilage and allow limited movement.
- **Synovial joints** allow for a range of motion and are covered by articular cartilage that protects the bones.

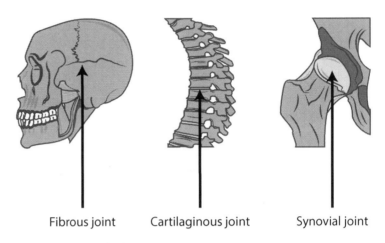

Fibrous joint   Cartilaginous joint   Synovial joint

Figure 7.15. Types of Joints

Synovial joints are classified based on their structure and the type of movement they allow. There are many types of synovial joints; the most important are discussed in Table 7.3.

TABLE 7.3. Types of Synovial Joints		
NAME	**MOVEMENT**	**FOUND IN**
Hinge joint	movement through one plane of motion as flexion/extension	elbows, knees, fingers
Ball-and-socket joint	range of motion through multiple planes and rotation about an axis	hips, shoulders
Saddle joint	movement through multiple planes, but cannot rotate about an axis	thumbs
Gliding joint	sliding movement in the plane of the bones' surfaces	vertebrae, small bones in the wrists and ankles
Condyloid joint	movement through two planes as flexion/extension and abduction/adduction, but cannot rotate about an axis	wrists
Pivot joint	only movement is rotation about an axis	elbows, neck

Pathologies of the Skeletal System

Arthritis is inflammation in joints that leads to swelling, pain, and reduced range of motion. There are many different kinds of arthritis. The most common is **osteoarthritis**, which is caused by the wearing down of cartilage in the joints due to age or injury. **Rheumatoid arthritis** and **psoriatic arthritis** are both types of inflammation at the joint caused by chronic autoimmune disorder, which can lead to excessive joint degradation.

Osteoporosis refers to poor bone mineral density due to the loss or lack of the production of calcium content and bone cells, which leads to bone brittleness. It is most common in postmenopausal women.

Bone cancers include Ewing's sarcoma and osteosarcoma. In addition, white blood cell cancers, such as myeloma and leukemia, start in bone marrow. **Osteomyelitis** is an infection in the bone that can occur directly (after a traumatic bone injury) or indirectly (via the vascular system or other infected tissues).

PRACTICE QUESTIONS

13. Stem cells are found in which of the following tissues?

    A) red bone marrow

    B) cartilage

    C) compact bones

    D) bone matrix

14. Which of the following parts of the skeletal system is formed from long bones?

    A) limbs

    B) thoracic cage

    C) skull

    D) vertebral column

15. Which of the following is released when bone is broken down?

    A) phosphorous

    B) iron

    C) calcium

    D) zinc

The Muscular System

The primary function of the muscular system is movement. Muscles contract and relax, resulting in motion. This includes both voluntary motion, such as walking, as well as involuntary motion that maintains the body's systems, such as circulation, respiration, and digestion. Other functions of the muscular system include overall stability and protection of the spine as well as posture.

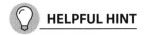
Muscle Cell Structure

The main structural unit of a muscle is the **sarcomere**. Sarcomeres are composed of thin filaments made of the protein **actin** and thick filaments made of the protein **myosin**. Each of these proteins plays a role in muscle contraction and relaxation. During muscle contractions, myosin pulls the thin filaments of actin to the center of the sarcomere, causing the entire sarcomere to shorten, or contract, creating movement. Bundles of these proteins are called **myofibrils**.

Skeletal muscles are activated by special neurons called **motor neurons**. Together, a motor neuron and its associated skeletal muscle fibers are called a **motor unit**. These motor neurons are located within the spinal cord and branch out to the muscles to send the nervous impulses for muscular contraction. The **neuromuscular junction** is the site at which the motor neuron and muscle fibers join to form a chemical synapse for nervous transmission to muscle.

Types of Muscles

The muscular system consists of three types of muscle: cardiac, visceral, and skeletal. **Cardiac muscle** is only found in the heart and contracts involuntarily, creating the heartbeat and pumping blood. **Visceral muscles** are found in many of the body's essential organs, including the stomach and intestines. They slowly contract and relax to move nutrients, blood, and other substances throughout the body. Visceral muscles are also known as **smooth muscles** because, unlike cardiac and skeletal muscle, this tissue is not composed of sarcomeres with alternating thick and thin filaments. Visceral muscle movement is involuntary.

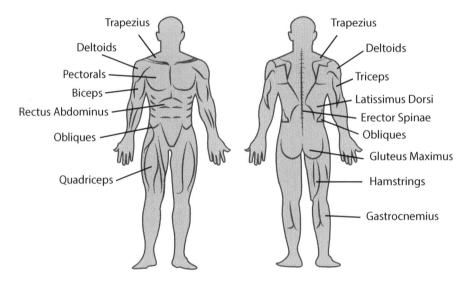

Figure 7.16. Major Muscles of the Body

Skeletal muscle is responsible for voluntary movement and, as the name suggests, is inextricably linked to the skeletal system. Skeletal muscles can engage in several types of muscle actions:

- **concentric**: muscular contraction in which the length of the muscle is shortening to lift the resistance (upward curl of bicep)

- **eccentric**: muscular contraction in which the muscle is resisting a force as it lengthens (downward curl of bicep)
- **isometric**: muscular contraction in which the resistance and force are even and no movement is taking place (holding an object)

Pathologies of the Muscular System

Injuries to muscle can impede movement and cause pain. When muscle fibers are overstretched, the resulting **muscle strain** can cause pain, stiffness, and bruising. Muscle **cramps** are involuntary muscle contractions (or **spasms**) that cause intense pain.

Muscle fibers can also be weakened by diseases, as with **muscular dystrophy (MD)**. MD is a genetically inherited condition that results in progressive muscle wasting, which limits movement and can cause respiratory and cardiovascular difficulties.

Rhabdomyolysis is the rapid breakdown of dead muscle tissue. It is usually caused by crush injuries, overexertion (particularly in extreme heat), and a variety of drugs and toxins (particularly statins, which are prescribed to lower cholesterol levels).

PRACTICE QUESTIONS

16. Which of the following types of muscle is found in blood vessels?

A) cardiac muscle

B) visceral muscle

C) type I muscle fibers

D) type II muscle fibers

17. Which of the following processes is performed by myofibrils?

A) sugar storage

B) electrochemical communication

C) lactic acid fermentation

D) muscle contractions

18. Which of the following causes a muscle strain?

A) a lack of available energy

B) the inability of muscle fibers to contract

C) detachment of the ligament from the bone

D) overstretching of muscle fibers

The Immune System

Structure and Function of the Immune System

The human immune system protects the body against bacteria and viruses that cause disease. The system is composed of two parts, the innate system and the adaptive system. The **innate immune system** includes nonspecific defenses that work against a wide range of infectious agents. This system includes both physical barriers that keep out foreign particles and organisms along with cells that attack invaders. The second part of the immune system is the **adaptive immune system**, which "learns" to respond only to specific invaders.

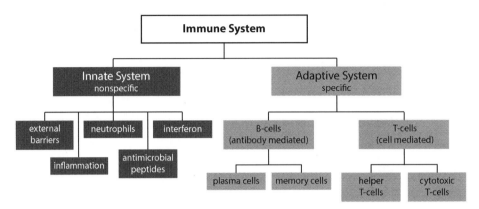

Figure 7.17. Divisions of the Immune System

Barriers to entry are the first line of defense in the immune system:

- The skin leaves few openings for an infection-causing agent to enter.
- Native bacteria outcompete invaders in openings.
- The urethra flushes out invaders with the outflow of urine.
- Mucus and earwax trap pathogens before they can replicate and cause infection.

However, pathogens can breach these barriers and enter the body, where they attempt to replicate and cause an infection. When this occurs, the body mounts a number of nonspecific responses. The body's initial response is **inflammation**, which increases blood flow to the infected area. This increase in blood flow increases the presence of white blood cells, also called **leukocytes**. (The types of white blood cells are discussed in Table 7.4.) Other innate responses include **antimicrobial peptides**, which destroy bacteria by interfering with the functions of their membranes or DNA, and **interferon**, which causes nearby cells to increase their defenses.

The adaptive immune system relies on molecules called **antigens** that appear on the surface of pathogens to which the system has previously been exposed. Antigens are displayed on the surface of cells by the **major histocompatibility complex (MHC)**.

In the cell-mediated response, **T-cells** destroy any cell that displays an antigen. In the antibody-mediated response, **B-cells** are activated by antigens. These B-cells produce plasma cells, which in turn release antibodies. **Antibodies** will bind only to specific antigens and destroy the infected cell. **Memory B-cells** are created during infection, allowing the immune system to respond more quickly if the infection appears again.

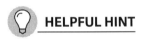 **HELPFUL HINT**

Memory B-cells are the underlying mechanisms behind vaccines, which introduce a harmless version of a pathogen into the body to activate the body's adaptive immune response.

TABLE 7.4. Types of White Blood Cells

TYPE OF CELL	NAME OF CELL	ROLE	INNATE OR ADAPTIVE	PREVALENCE
Granulocytes	neutrophil	first responders that quickly migrate to the site of infections to destroy bacterial invaders	innate	very common
	eosinophil	attack multicellular parasites	innate	rare
	basophil	large cell responsible for inflammatory reactions, including allergies	innate	very rare
Lymphocytes	B-cells	respond to antigens by releasing antibodies	adaptive	common
	T-cells	respond to antigens by destroying invaders and infected cells	adaptive	
	natural killer cells	destroy virus-infected cells and tumor cells	innate and adaptive	
Monocytes	macrophage	engulf and destroy microbes, foreign substances, and cancer cells	innate and adaptive	rare

Pathologies of the Immune System

The immune system of individuals with an **autoimmune disease** will attack healthy tissues. Autoimmune diseases (and the tissues they attack) include:

- psoriasis (skin)
- rheumatoid arthritis (joints)
- multiple sclerosis (nerve cells)
- lupus (kidneys, lungs, and skin)

The immune system may also overreact to harmless particles, a condition known as an **allergy**. Allergic reactions can be mild, resulting in watery eyes and a runny nose, but they can also include life-threatening swelling and respiratory obstruction.

Some infections will attack the immune system itself. **Human immunodeficiency virus (HIV)** attacks helper T-cells, eventually causing **acquired immunodeficiency syndrome (AIDS)**, which allows opportunistic infections to overrun the body. The immune system can also be weakened by previous infections or lifestyle factors such as smoking and alcohol consumption.

Cancers of the immune system include **lymphoma** and **leukemia**, which are caused by irregular growth of cells in lymph and bone marrow. Both white and red blood cells can become cancerous, but it is more common for the cancer to occur in white blood cells. Leukemia is the most common type of cancer to occur in children.

PRACTICE QUESTIONS

19. Which of the following is NOT part of the innate immune system?

    A) interferon

    B) neutrophils

    C) antibodies

    D) natural killer lymphocytes

20. Which of the following is a response by the innate immune system when tissue is damaged?

    A) The skin dries out.

    B) The temperature increases.

    C) The blood flow to the area decreases.

    D) The heart rate slows.

21. What is the role of monocytes in wounds?

    A) They increase blood clotting.

    B) They release histamines.

    C) They digest pathogens.

    D) They prevent inflammation.

The Digestive System

Structure and Function of the Digestive System

The **digestive system** is responsible for the breakdown and absorption of food necessary to power the body. The digestive system starts at the **mouth**, which allows for the consumption and mastication of nutrients via an opening in the face. It contains the muscular **tongue** to move food and uses the liquid **saliva** to assist in the breakdown of food.

The chewed and lubricated food travels from the mouth through the **esophagus** via **peristalsis**, the contraction of smooth muscles. The esophagus leads to the **stomach**, the organ of the digestive tract found in the abdominal cavity that mixes food with powerful acidic liquid for further digestion. Once the stomach has created an acidic bolus of digested food known as **chyme**, it travels to the **small intestine**, where a significant amount of nutrient absorption takes place. The tubelike small intestine contains millions of fingerlike projections known as **villi** and microvilli to increase the surface area available for the absorption of nutrients found in food.

The small intestine then transports food to the **large intestine**. The large intestine is similarly tubelike but is larger in diameter than the small intestine. It assists in water absorption, further nutrient absorption, waste collection, and the production of feces for excretion. At the end of the large intestine are the **rectum** and the **anus**, which are responsible for the storage of feces and removal of feces, respectively. The anus is the opening at the opposite end of the digestive tract as the mouth.

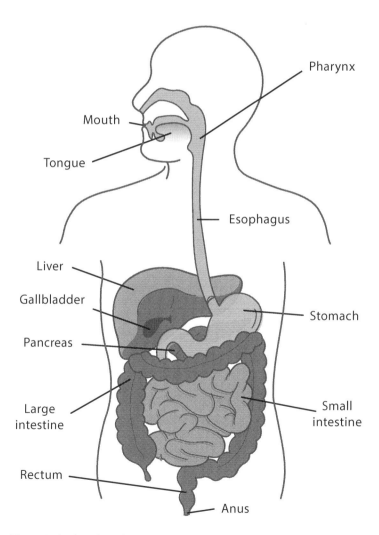

Figure 7.18. The Digestive System

 HELPFUL HINT

Digestive enzymes work through the GI tract to break down macromolecules to be used in bodily processes.

amylase: breaks down carbohydrates in the mouth

lipase: breaks down lipids in the mouth

pepsin: breaks down proteins in the stomach

lactase: breaks down lactose in the small intestine

protease: breaks down proteins in the small intestine

Along the digestive tract are several muscular rings, known as **sphincters**, which regulate the movement of food through the tract and prevent reflux of material into the previous cavity. These include:

- upper esophageal sphincter: between the pharynx and esophagus
- lower esophageal sphincter: between the esophagus and stomach
- pyloric sphincter: between the stomach and small intestine
- ileocecal sphincter: between the small intestine and large intestine
- anus: between the rectum and the outside of the body

The digestive system also includes accessory organs that aid in digestion:

- **salivary glands**: produce saliva, which begins the process of breaking down starches and fats
- **liver**: produces bile, which helps break down fat in the small intestine
- **gallbladder**: stores bile
- **pancreas**: produces digestive enzymes and pancreatic juice, which neutralizes the acidity of chyme

Pathologies of the Digestive System

The digestive system is prone to several illnesses of varying severity. Commonly, gastrointestinal distress is caused by an acute infection (bacterial or viral) affecting the lining of the digestive system that leads to vomiting and diarrhea.

Chronic GI disorders include **irritable bowel syndrome** (the causes of which are largely unknown) and **Crohn's disease**, an inflammatory bowel disorder that occurs when the immune system attacks the digestive system.

A number of different cancers can arise in the digestive system, including colon and rectal cancer, liver cancer, pancreatic cancer, esophageal cancer, and stomach cancer. Of these, colon cancer is the most common.

 DID YOU KNOW?

The veins of the stomach and intestines do not carry blood directly to the heart. Instead, they divert it to the liver (through the **hepatic portal vein**) so that the liver can store sugar, remove toxins, and process the products of digestion.

PRACTICE QUESTIONS

22. Which of the following organs does food NOT pass through as part of digestion?

    A) stomach

    B) large intestine

    C) esophagus

    D) liver

23. Where in the digestive tract are most of the nutrients absorbed?

    A) the small intestine

    B) the rectum

    C) the stomach

    D) the large intestine

24. What is the role of the liver in digestion?

A) It produces the bile needed to digest fats.

B) It stores bile produced by the gallbladder.

C) It regulates feelings of hunger.

D) It collects the waste that is the end product of digestion.

The Urinary System

Structure and Function of the Urinary System

The **urinary system** excretes water and waste from the body and is crucial for maintaining the balance of water and salt in the blood (also called electrolyte balance). Because many organs function as part of both the reproductive and urinary systems, the two are sometimes referred to collectively as the **genitourinary system**.

The main organs of the urinary system are the **kidneys**, which perform several important functions:

- filter waste from the blood
- maintain the electrolyte balance in the blood
- regulate blood volume, pressure, and pH

The kidneys also function as an endocrine organ and release several important hormones, including **renin**, which regulates blood pressure. The kidney is divided into two regions: the **renal cortex**, which is the outermost layer, and the **renal medulla**, which is the inner layer.

The functional unit of the kidney is the **nephron**, which is a series of looping tubes that filter the blood. The resulting waste includes **urea**, a byproduct of protein catabolism, and **uric acid**, a byproduct of

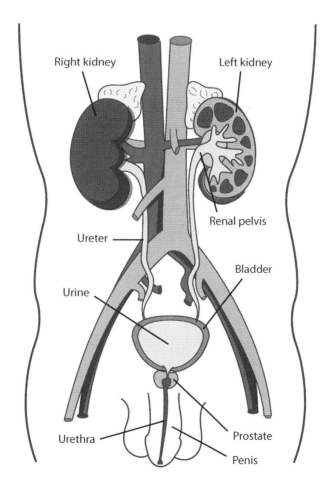

Figure 7.19. The Urinary System (Male)

nucleic acid metabolism. Together, these waste products are excreted from the body in **urine**.

Filtration begins in a network of capillaries called a **glomerulus**, which is located in the renal cortex of each kidney. This waste is then funneled into **collecting ducts** in the renal medulla. From the collecting ducts, urine passes through the **renal pelvis** and then through two long tubes called **ureters**. The two ureters drain into the **urinary bladder**, which holds up to 1 liter of liquid. Urine exits the bladder through the **urethra**. In males, the urethra goes through the penis and also carries semen. In females, the much-shorter urethra ends just above the vaginal opening.

Pathologies of the Urinary System

Urinary tract infections (UTIs) occur when bacteria infects the kidneys, bladder, or urethra. They can occur in men or women but are more common in women. **Pyelonephritis**, infection of the kidneys, occurs when bacteria reach the kidneys via the lower urinary tract or the bloodstream.

Chronic kidney disease, in which the kidneys do not function properly for at least three months, can be caused by a number of factors, including diabetes, autoimmune diseases, infections, and drug abuse. People with chronic kidney disease may need **dialysis**, during which a machine performs the task of the kidneys and removes waste from the blood.

Renal calculi (kidney stones) are hardened mineral deposits that form in the kidneys. They are usually asymptomatic but will cause debilitating pain and urinary symptoms once they pass into the urinary tract.

PRACTICE QUESTIONS

25. Which of the following is the outermost layer of the kidney?
    A) renal cortex
    B) renal medulla
    C) renal pelvis
    D) nephron

26. Which of the following organs holds urine before it passes into the urethra?
    A) prostate
    B) kidney
    C) ureter
    D) urinary bladder

The Reproductive System

The Male Reproductive System

The **male reproductive system** produces **sperm**, or male gametes, and passes them to the female reproductive system. Sperm are produced during spermatogenesis in the **testes** (also called testicles), which are housed in a sac-like external structure called the **scrotum**. The scrotum contracts and relaxes to move the testes closer to or farther from the body. This process keeps the testes at the appropriate temperature for sperm production, which is slightly lower than regular body temperature.

Mature sperm are stored in the **epididymis**. During sexual stimulation, sperm travel from the epididymis through a long, thin tube called the **vas deferens**. Along the way, the sperm are joined by fluids from three glands:

- The **seminal vesicles** secrete a fluid composed of various proteins, sugars, and enzymes.

- The **prostate** contributes an alkaline fluid that counteracts the acidity of the vaginal tract.

- The **Cowper's gland** secretes a protein-rich fluid that acts as a lubricant.

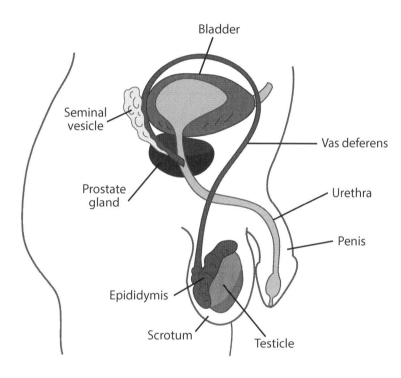

Figure 7.20. The Male Reproductive System

The mix of fluids and sperm, called **semen**, travels through the **urethra** and exits the body through the **penis**, which becomes rigid during sexual arousal.

The main hormone associated with the male reproductive system is **testosterone**, which is released by the testes (and in the adrenal glands in much smaller amounts). Testosterone is responsible for the development of the male reproductive system and male secondary sexual characteristics, including muscle development and facial hair growth.

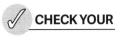 CHECK YOUR

UNDERSTANDING

What type of muscle is most likely found in the myometrium of the uterus?

The Female Reproductive System

The female reproductive system produces **eggs**, or female gametes, and gestates the fetus during pregnancy. Eggs are produced in the **ovaries** and travel through the **fallopian tubes** to the **uterus**, which is a muscular organ that houses the fetus during pregnancy. The uterine cavity is lined with a layer of blood-rich tissue called the **endometrium**. If no pregnancy occurs, the endometrium is shed monthly during **menstruation**.

Fertilization occurs when the egg absorbs the sperm; it usually takes place in the fallopian tubes but may happen in the uterus itself. After fertilization the new zygote implants itself in the endometrium, where it will grow and develop over thirty-eight weeks (roughly nine months). During gestation, the developing fetus acquires nutrients and passes waste through the **placenta**. This temporary organ is attached to the wall of the uterus and is connected to the baby by the **umbilical cord**.

When the fetus is mature, powerful muscle contractions occur in the **myometrium**, the muscular layer next to the endometrium. These contractions push the fetus through an opening called the **cervix** into the **vagina**, from which the fetus exits the body. The placenta and umbilical cords are also expelled through the vagina shortly after birth.

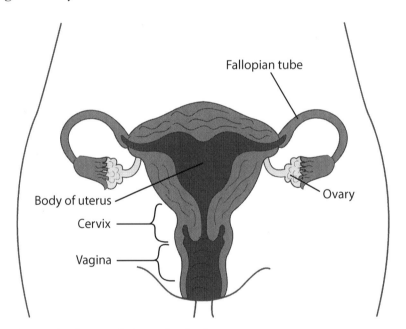

Figure 7.21. The Female Reproductive System

The female reproductive cycle is controlled by a number of different hormones. **Estrogen**, produced by the ovaries, stimulates Graafian follicles, which contain immature egg cells. The pituitary gland then releases **luteinizing hormone**, which causes the egg to be released into the fallopian tube during ovulation. During pregnancy, estrogen and **progesterone** are released in high levels to help with fetal growth and to prevent further ovulation.

Pathologies of the Reproductive System

Sexually transmitted infections (STIs) include **chlamydia, gonorrhea, human papillomavirus (HPV),** and **genital herpes**. Both chlamydia and gonorrhea are bacterial infections that have few symptoms in men but can cause burning, itching, and discharge in women. HPV and genital herpes are both viral infections that lead to warts and open sores, respectively. HPV has also been linked to the development of cervical cancer.

When untreated, bacterial infections in the female reproductive system can lead to **pelvic inflammatory disease (PID)**. Symptoms of PID include abdominal pain, fever, and vaginal discharge. PID is one of the most common causes of infertility.

Endometriosis is a condition in which endometrial tissue, which usually lines the inside of the uterus, grows outside the uterus. Symptoms include pain, irregular or painful menstruation, and infertility.

Cancers of the female reproductive system include ovarian cancer, cervical cancer, and uterine cancer. **Prostate cancer** is a common but slow-growing cancer of the male reproductive system. It is most common in patients over fifty.

PRACTICE QUESTIONS

27. Which of the following organs does NOT contribute material to semen?

   A) the prostate

   B) the Cowper's glands

   C) the penis

   D) the testes

28. Fertilization typically takes place in the

   A) fallopian tube.

   B) ovaries.

   C) uterus.

   D) cervix.

The Endocrine System

Structure and Function of the Endocrine System

The endocrine system is made up of **glands** that regulate numerous processes throughout the body by secreting chemical messengers called **hormones**. These hormones regulate a wide variety of bodily processes, including metabolism, growth and development, sexual reproduction, the sleep-wake cycle, and hunger.

The **hypothalamus** is a gland that plays a central role in the endocrine system by connecting it to the nervous system. Input from the nervous system reaches the hypothalamus, causing it to release hormones from the **pituitary gland**. These hormones in turn regulate the release of hormones from many of the other endocrine glands.

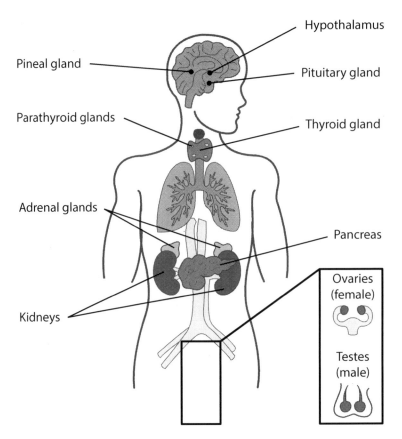

Figure 7.22. The Location of Endocrine Glands

TABLE 7.5. Endocrine Glands and Their Functions		
GLAND	**REGULATES**	**HORMONES PRODUCED**
Hypothalamus	pituitary function and metabolic processes including body temperature, hunger, thirst, and circadian rhythms	thyrotropin-releasing hormone (TRH), dopamine, growth hormone–releasing hormone (GHRH), gonadotropin-releasing hormone (GnRH), oxytocin, vasopressin
Pituitary gland	growth, blood pressure, reabsorption of water by the kidneys, temperature, pain relief, and some reproductive functions related to pregnancy and childbirth	human growth hormone (HGH), thyroid-stimulating hormone (TSH), prolactin (PRL), luteinizing hormone (LH), follicle-stimulating hormone (FSH), oxytocin, antidiuretic hormone (ADH)
Pineal gland	circadian rhythms (the sleep-wake cycle)	melatonin
Thyroid gland	energy use and protein synthesis	thyroxine (T_4), triiodothyronine (T_3), calcitonin
Parathyroid	calcium and phosphate levels	parathyroid hormone (PTH)

GLAND	REGULATES	HORMONES PRODUCED
Adrenal glands	fight-or-flight response and regulation of salt and blood volume	epinephrine, norepinephrine, cortisol, androgens
Pancreas	blood sugar levels and metabolism	insulin, glucagon, somatostatin
Testes	maturation of sex organs, and secondary sex characteristics	androgens (e.g., testosterone)
Ovaries	maturation of sex organs, secondary sex characteristics, pregnancy, childbirth, and lactation	progesterone, estrogen
Placenta	gestation and childbirth	progesterone, estrogen, human chorionic gonadotropin, human placental lactogen (hPL)

Many important hormones can be broken down into either anabolic hormones or catabolic hormones. **Anabolic hormones** are associated with the regulation of growth and development; these include testosterone, estrogen, insulin, and human growth hormone. **Human growth hormone** is released by the pituitary gland and regulates muscle and bone development. Another example of an anabolic hormone is **insulin-like growth factor (IGF)**, which is synthesized in the liver and aids in tissue growth and many other functions. **Catabolic hormones** help regulate the breakdown of substances into smaller molecules. For example, the breakdown of muscle glycogen for energy via the release of **glucagon** is a catabolic process.

Pathologies of the Endocrine System

Disruption of hormone production in specific endocrine glands can lead to disease. Overactive or underactive glands can lead to conditions like **hypothyroidism**, which is characterized by a slow metabolism, and **hyperparathyroidism**, which can lead to osteoporosis. **Adrenal insufficiency** (Addison's disease) is the chronic underproduction of steroids.

Diabetes mellitus is a metabolic disorder that affects the body's ability to produce and use **insulin**, a hormone that regulates cellular uptake of glucose (sugar).

- Uncontrolled diabetes can lead to high blood glucose levels (**hyperglycemia**) or low blood glucose levels (**hypoglycemia**).

- **Type 1 diabetes** is an acute-onset autoimmune disease predominant in children, teens, and adults under 30. Beta cells in the pancreas are destroyed and are unable to produce sufficient amounts of insulin, causing blood glucose to rise.

 DID YOU KNOW?

One of the most prescribed medications in the United States is levothyroxine (Synthroid), a manufactured form of the hormone thyroxine. It is prescribed for patients with underactive thyroids.

 DID YOU KNOW?

More than 30 million Americans have been diagnosed with diabetes. In the United States, more money is spent on health care related to diabetes than on any other single medical condition.

- **Type 2 diabetes** is a gradual-onset disease predominant in adults under 40, but it can develop in individuals of all ages. The person develops insulin resistance, which prevents the cellular uptake of glucose and causes blood glucose to rise. Type 2 diabetes accounts for 90% of all diabetes diagnoses in the United States.

- Diabetes requires long-term management with insulin or oral hypoglycemic drugs.

Thyroid cancer is relatively common but has few or no symptoms. In addition, benign (noncancerous) tumors on the thyroid and other endocrine glands can damage the functioning of a wide variety of bodily systems.

PRACTICE QUESTIONS

29. Which of the following glands indirectly controls growth by acting on the pituitary gland?

A) hypothalamus

B) thyroid gland

C) adrenal glands

D) parathyroid glands

30. A patient experiencing symptoms such as kidney stones and arthritis due to a calcium imbalance probably has a disorder of which of the following glands?

A) hypothalamus

B) thyroid gland

C) parathyroid glands

D) adrenal glands

The Integumentary System

Structure and Function of the Integumentary System

The **integumentary system** refers to the skin (the largest organ in the body) and related structures, including the hair and nails. Skin is composed of three layers. The **epidermis** is the outermost layer of the skin. This waterproof layer contains no blood vessels and acts mainly to protect the body. Under the epidermis lies the **dermis**, which consists of dense connective tissue that allows skin to stretch and flex. The dermis is home to blood vessels, glands, and hair follicles. The **hypodermis** is a layer of fat below the dermis that stores energy (in the form of fat) and acts as a cushion for the body. The hypodermis is sometimes called the **subcutaneous layer**.

The skin has several important roles. It acts as a barrier to protect the body from injury, the intrusion of foreign particles, and the loss of water and nutrients. It is also important for **thermoregulation**. Blood vessels near the surface of the skin can dilate, allowing for higher blood flow and the release of heat. They can also constrict to reduce the amount of blood that travels near the surface of the skin, which helps conserve heat. In addition, the skin produces **vitamin D** when exposed to sunlight.

Because the skin covers the whole body, it plays a vital role in allowing organisms to interact with the environment. It is home to nerve endings that sense temperature, pressure, and pain, and it also houses glands that help maintain homeostasis. **Eccrine glands**, which are located primarily in the palms of the hands and soles of the feet (and to a lesser degree in other areas of the body), release the water and salt mixture (sodium chloride, NaCl) called **sweat**. These glands help the body maintain the appropriate salt-water balance. Sweat can also contain small amounts of other substances the body needs to expel, including alcohol, lactic acid, and urea.

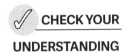

CHECK YOUR UNDERSTANDING

Why would flushing—the reddening of the skin caused by dilating blood vessels—be associated with fevers?

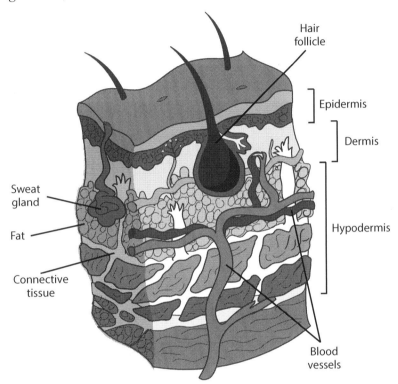

Figure 7.23. The Skin

Apocrine glands, which are located primarily in the armpit and groin, release an oily substance that contains pheromones. They are also sensitive to adrenaline and are responsible for most of the sweating that occurs due to stress, fear, anxiety, or pain. Apocrine glands are largely inactive until puberty.

Pathologies of the Integumentary System

Psoriasis is an autoimmune condition that causes inflammation in the skin, resulting in red, flaking patches on the skin. **Eczema** (atopic dermatitis) is a red, itchy rash that usually occurs in children but can occur in adults as well.

Skin cancers can be categorized as melanoma or nonmelanoma cancers. **Melanoma** cancers appear as irregular, dark patches on the skin and are more difficult to treat than nonmelanoma cancers.

PRACTICE QUESTIONS

31. Which of the following is NOT a function of the skin?

   A) regulating body temperature

   B) protecting against injury

   C) producing adrenaline

   D) maintaining water-salt balance

32. Which of the following is the outermost layer of the skin?

   A) hypodermis

   B) dermis

   C) epidermis

   D) apocrine

Homeostasis

The human body has many complex systems that maintain **homeostasis**—the body's internal equilibrium. These processes allow the body to monitor external changes and adapt by altering body temperature, blood sugar, blood pressure, and other physiological states.

Feedback mechanisms are the primary forms of communication between the systems working to maintain homeostasis. In a **negative feedback loop**, an external change prompts a response to return the body's internal environmental back to equilibrium. For example, if exposure to heat causes the body's internal temperature to rise, the body will attempt to cool down. Receptors in the skin detect the change in temperature and relay the message to the hypothalamus, which signals sweat glands to release sweat, cooling the body. The **process** of maintaining homeostasis of internal body temperature is known as **thermoregulation**.

Another example of a negative feedback loop is the regulation of blood glucose levels. When food is consumed, blood glucose levels rise. This rise stimulates the pancreas to produce **insulin**, a hormone that moves glucose into cells, reducing blood glucose levels. When blood glucose is low, the pancreas secretes **glucagon**, a hormone that stimulates production of glucose in the liver. Together, these hormones keep blood glucose in a normal, healthy range.

Positive feedback loops are not used to maintain homeostasis; instead, they exacerbate the initial response to a stimulus. Positive feedback loops in the body are rare. One example is the release of oxytocin during childbirth. During labor, the pressure of the fetus on the cervix triggers the release of **oxytocin**, which stimulates uterine contractions. The contractions further increase the pressure on the cervix, resulting in the release of more oxytocin. This cycle continues until the baby is born.

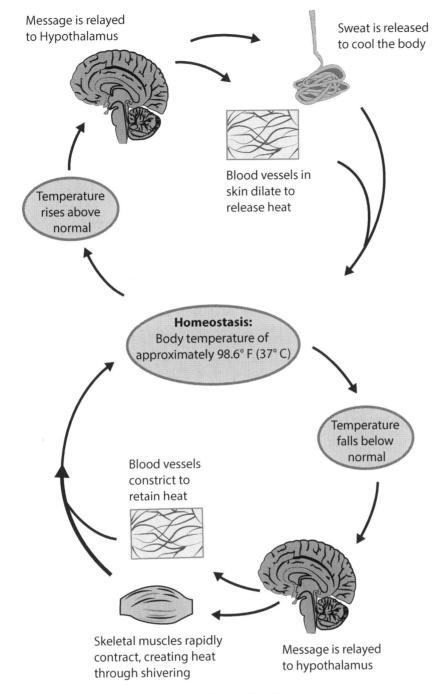

Figure 7.24. Negative Thermoregulation Feedback Loop

PRACTICE QUESTION

33. Which of the following hormones is replaced when blood glucose levels in the body are too high?

   A) insulin

   B) oxytocin

   C) glucagon

   D) thyroxine

Answer Key

1. **A)** The meninges are connective tissue.

2. **A)** The wrist is distal, or farther from the trunk, relative to the elbow.

3. **C)** The abdominal cavity holds organs involved in urinary and digestive function, including the appendix.

4. **A)** The myocardium is the muscular layer of the heart that contains cardiac muscle.

5. **D)** The right ventricle pumps deoxygenated blood from the heart to the lungs.

6. **D)** Blood leaves the heart in arteries.

7. **D)** The epiglottis covers the esophagus during respiration so that air does not enter the digestive track.

8. **C)** The alveoli are sacs found at the terminal end of each bronchiole in the lungs and are the site of gas exchange with the blood.

9. **C)** Asthma is a negative reaction of the body to otherwise harmless particles.

10. **B)** The axon carries information away from the soma, or body of the cell.

11. **B)** The somatic nervous system controls voluntary actions.

12. **A)** Schwann cells secrete myelin, which forms a sheet around the neuron and allows the electrical signal to travel faster.

13. **A)** Stem cells are found in red bone marrow.

14. **A)** Long bones are the main bones composing the arms and legs.

15. **C)** Calcium is released as bones are degraded, which helps balance the calcium level in the body.

16. **B)** Blood is moved through blood vessels by visceral, or smooth, muscle that cannot be voluntarily controlled.

17. **D)** Myofibrils are the muscle fibers that contract.

18. **D)** A muscle strain is caused by the overstretching of muscle fibers, resulting in tearing of the muscle.

19. **C)** Antibodies are part of the body's adaptive immune system and only respond to specific pathogens.

20. **B)** Inflammation increases the blood flow to the damaged area, increasing its temperature and bringing white blood cells to the site.

21. **C)** Monocytes use phagocytosis to "swallow" and break down pathogens.

22. **D)** The liver is an accessory organ of the digestive system: it produces fluids that aid in digestion, but food does not pass through it.

23. **A)** Most nutrients are absorbed by the small intestine.

24. **A)** The liver produces bile, which is needed for the digestion of fats.

25. **A)** The outermost layer of the kidney is the renal cortex.

26. **D)** The urinary bladder holds urine before it passes to the urethra to be excreted.

27. **C)** Semen travels through the penis to exit the body, but the penis does not itself produce any material to contribute to semen.

28. **A)** Fertilization takes place when a sperm enters an egg in the fallopian tube.

29. **A)** The hypothalamus releases hormones that in turn cause the pituitary gland to release growth-related hormones.

30. **C)** The parathyroid glands regulate levels of calcium and phosphate in the body.

31. **C)** The skin does not produce adrenaline. (Adrenaline is produced and released by the adrenal glands.)

32. **C)** The epidermis is the outermost layer of the skin. It is waterproof and does not contain any blood vessels.

33. **A)** When blood glucose levels rise, the body releases insulin to move glucose into cells and lower blood glucose levels.

8 | Biology

Biological Macromolecules

Organic and Inorganic Compounds

Organic compounds are those that contain carbon. These compounds, such as glucose, triacylglycerol, and guanine, are used in day-to-day metabolic processes. Many of these molecules are **polymers** formed from repeated smaller units called **monomers**. **Inorganic** compounds are those that do not contain carbon. These make up a very small fraction of mass in living organisms and are usually minerals such as potassium, sodium, and iron.

There are several classes of organic compounds commonly found in living organisms. These biological molecules include carbohydrates, proteins, lipids, and nucleic acids, which, when combined, make up more than 95 percent of non-water material in living organisms.

PRACTICE QUESTION

1. Organic molecules must contain which element?

    A) carbon

    B) phosphorous

    C) nitrogen

    D) oxygen

Carbohydrates

Carbohydrates, also called sugars, are molecules made of carbon, hydrogen, and oxygen. Sugars are primarily used in organisms as a source of energy: they can be catabolized (broken down) to create energy molecules such as adenosine triphosphate (ATP) or nicotinamide adenine dinucleotide (NAD^+), providing a source of electrons to drive cellular processes.

The monomer of carbohydrates is the **monosaccharide**, a sugar with the formula $C_nH_{2n}O_n$. Glucose, for example, is the monosaccharide $C_6H_{12}O_6$. Simple sugars like glucose can bond together to form polymers called **polysaccharides**. Some polymers of glucose include starch, which is used to store excess sugar, and cellulose, which is a support fiber responsible in part for the strength of plants.

Glucose: $C_6H_{12}O_6$

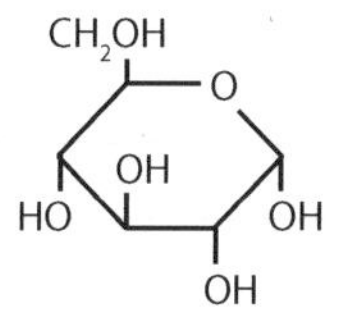

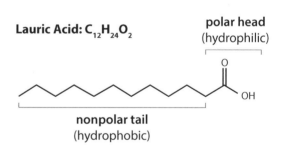

Figure 8.1. A Carbohydrate

PRACTICE QUESTION

2. Which of the following compounds is NOT created by joining monosaccharides?

   A) glycogen

   B) starch

   C) cellulose

   D) guanine

Lipids

Lipids are compounds primarily composed of carbon and hydrogen with only a small percentage of oxygen. Lipids contain a **head**, usually formed of glycerol or phosphate, and a **tail**, which is a hydrocarbon chain. The composition of the head, whether it is a carboxylic acid functional group, a phosphate group, or some other functional group, is usually polar, meaning it is hydrophilic. The tail is composed of carbon and hydrogen and is usually nonpolar, meaning it is hydrophobic.

The combined polarity of the lipid head and the non-polarity of the lipid tail are unique features of lipids critical to the formation of the phospholipid bilayer in the cell membrane. The fatty acid tails all point inward, and the heads point outward. This provides a semipermeable membrane that allows a cell to separate its contents from the environment.

Lauric Acid: $C_{12}H_{24}O_2$

polar head (hydrophilic)

nonpolar tail (hydrophobic)

Figure 8.2. A Lipid (Lauric Acid)

The **saturation** of a lipid describes the number of double bonds in the tail of the lipid. The more double bonds a lipid tail has, the more unsaturated the molecule is, and the more bends there are in its structure. As a result, unsaturated fats (like oils) tend to be liquid at room temperature, whereas saturated fats (like lard or butter) are solid at room temperature.

3. The head of a lipid is composed of which molecule?

    A) glycerol

    B) glucose

    C) phospholipid

    D) cellulose

Proteins

Proteins are large molecules that play an important role in almost every cellular process in the human body. They act as catalysts, transport molecules across membranes, facilitate DNA replication, and regulate the cell cycle, including mitosis and meiosis.

Proteins are composed of a chain of **amino acids**. The sequence of amino acids in the chain determines the protein's structure and function. Each amino acid is composed of three parts:

- Amino group ($-NH_2$): The amino group is found on all amino acids.
- Carboxyl group ($-COOH$): The carboxyl group is found on all amino acids.
- R group: The R group is a unique functional group that is different for each amino acid.

There are twenty-two amino acids used to produce proteins. It is not necessary to know each amino acid, but it is important to know that sequences of these amino acids form proteins, and each amino acid has a unique R-functional group.

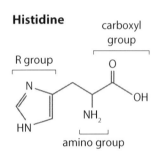

Figure 8.3. An Amino Acid (Histidine)

4. Proteins are built from monomers called

    A) carboxylic acids.

    B) nitrogenous bases.

    C) nucleic acids.

    D) amino acids.

Nucleic Acids

Nucleic acids, which include DNA and RNA, store all information necessary to produce proteins. These molecules are built using smaller molecules called **nucleotides**, which are composed of a 5-carbon sugar, a phosphate group, and a nitrogenous base.

DNA is made from four nucleotides: adenine, guanine, cytosine, and thymine. Together, adenine and guanine are classified as **purines**, while thymine and cytosine are classified as **pyrimidines**. These nucleotides bond together in pairs; the pairs are then bonded together in a chain to create a double helix shape with the sugar as the outside and the nitrogenous base on the inside. In DNA, adenine and thymine always bond together, as do guanine and cytosine. In RNA, thymine is replaced by a nucleotide called uracil, which bonds with adenine. RNA also differs from DNA in that it often exists as a single strand.

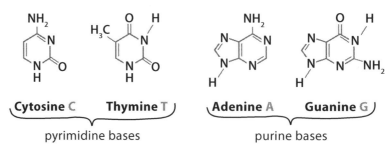

pyrimidine bases   purine bases

Figure 8.4. DNA Nucleotides

The individual strands of DNA are directional, meaning it matters in which direction the DNA is read. The two ends of a DNA strand are called the 3' end and the 5' end, and these names are included when describing a section of DNA, as shown below:

5'-ATGAATTGCCT-3'

For two complementary strands of DNA, one end starts at 5', and the other starts at 3':

5'-ATGAATTGCCT-3'
3'-TACTTAACGGA-5'

This naming convention is needed to understand the direction of DNA replication and where the enzymes bind during the process.

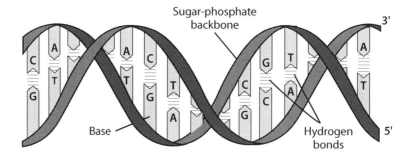

Figure 8.5. DNA Double Helix

PRACTICE QUESTIONS

5. Which of the following nucleotides is NOT found in DNA?

    A) adenine

    B) uracil

C) thymine

D) cytosine

6. Which of the following sequences is the complementary segment of this section of DNA: 5' AAGCCCTATAC 3'?

   A) 3' UUCGGGAUAUG 5'

   B) 3' TTCGGGATATG 5'

   C) 3' GTATAGGGCTT 5'

   D) 3' GUAUAGGGCUU 5'

Nucleic Acids

The Structure of DNA

A cell has a lot of DNA: even the smallest human cell contains a copy of the entire human genome. In human cells, this copy of the genome is nearly two meters in length—quite long, considering the average cell is only 100 µm in diameter.

In the nucleus, DNA is organized around proteins called **histones**; together, this protein and DNA complex is known as **chromatin**. During interphase, chromatin is usually arranged loosely to allow access to DNA. During mitosis, however, DNA is tightly packaged into units called **chromosomes**. When DNA has replicated, the chromosome is composed of two **chromatids** joined together at the **centromere**.

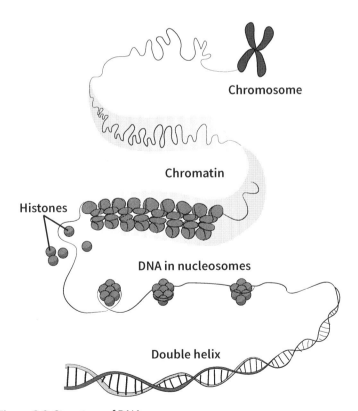

Figure 8.6. Structure of DNA

Each somatic cell is **diploid** (2*n*), meaning it has two sets of homologous chromosomes, one from each parent. For example, humans have twenty-three pairs of chromosomes, for a total of forty-six chromosomes. Gametes (sex cells) have only one set of chromosomes, so a human sex cell has twenty-three chromosomes. Cells with one set of chromosomes are referred to as **haploid** (1*n*).

PRACTICE QUESTION

7. To form nucleosomes, DNA is wrapped around

A) histones.

B) chromatin.

C) centromeres.

D) ATP.

DNA Replication

DNA replication is the process by which a copy of DNA is created in a cell. During DNA replication, three steps will occur. The first step is **initiation**, in which an initiator protein binds to regions of DNA known as origin sites. Once the initiation protein has been bound, the DNA polymerase complex will be able to attach. At this point, the enzyme helicase unwinds DNA into two separate single strands.

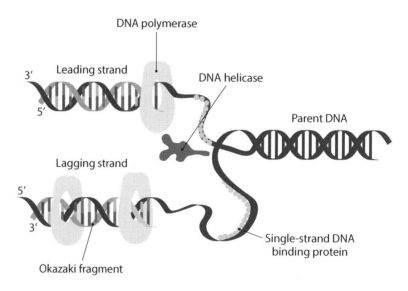

Figure 8.7. DNA replication

During the next step, **elongation**, new strands of DNA are created. Single-strand binding proteins (SSBs) will bind to each strand of the DNA. Then, DNA polymerase will attach and start replicating the strands by synthesizing a new, complementary strand. DNA polymerase reads the DNA in the 3' to 5' direction, meaning the new strand is synthesized in the 5' to 3' direction. This creates a problem, because the DNA can only be read in the 3' to 5' direction on one strand, known as the **leading strand**. The **lagging strand**, which runs from 5' to 3', has to be synthesized piece by piece in chunks called **Okazaki fragments**. The breaks between these fragments are later filled in by DNA ligase.

The last step in the process of DNA replication is **termination**. After DNA polymerase completes the copying process, the replication forks meet, and the process is terminated. There is one catch to this: because the DNA polymerase enzyme can never read or replicate the very end of a strand of DNA, every time a full chromosome is replicated, a small part of DNA is lost at the end. This piece of DNA is usually noncoding and is called a **telomere**. The shortening of the telomeres is the reason why replication can occur only a limited number of times in somatic cells before DNA replication is no longer possible.

TABLE 8.1. Important Enzymes in DNA Replication	
DNA Helicase	This unwinds a section of DNA to create a segment with two single strands.
DNA Polymerase	DNA polymerase I is responsible for synthesizing Okazaki fragments. DNA polymerase III is responsible for the primary replication of the 5' to 3' strand.
DNA Ligase	Ligase fixes small breaks in the DNA strand and is used to seal the finished DNA strands.
DNA Telomerase	In some cells, DNA telomerase lengthens the telomeres at the end of each strand of DNA, allowing it to be copied additional times.

PRACTICE QUESTIONS

8. Which of the following describes why small sections of DNA are lost during replication?

    A) The sections of DNA between Okazaki fragments cannot be recovered.

    B) DNA polymerase cannot replicate the end of the DNA strand.

    C) DNA cannot be read in the 5' to 3' direction.

    D) The initiator proteins bind to only one strand of DNA.

9. Which of the following is the enzyme that joins strands of DNA?

    A) DNA polymerase

    B) DNA telomerase

    C) DNA ligase

    D) DNA helicase

Transcription and Translation

The "message" contained in DNA and RNA is encoded in the nucleotides. Each amino acid is represented by a set of three base pairs in the nucleotide sequence called a **codon**. There are sixty-four possible codons (4 × 4 × 4), which means many of the twenty-two amino acids are coded for with more than one codon.

There are also three stop codons, which instruct the ribosome to stop processing the mRNA.

The processing of information stored in DNA to produce a protein takes place in two stages: transcription and translation. In transcription, an mRNA copy of the DNA is created. In translation, the mRNA strand is read by a ribosome to create an amino acid chain, which is folded into a protein.

DNA **transcription** is the process of making messenger RNA (mRNA) from a DNA strand. The steps for DNA transcription are similar to those of DNA replication, although different enzymes are used. The DNA strand provides a template for RNA polymerase: the DNA is first unwound, and then RNA polymerase makes a complementary transcript of the DNA sequence, called mRNA.

The **translation** process converts the mRNA transcript into a useable protein. This process occurs in a ribosome, which lines up the mRNA so it can bind to the appropriate tRNA (transfer RNA). Each tRNA includes an amino acid and an **anticodon**, which matches to the complementary codon on the mRNA. When the tRNA is in place, a bond is formed between the growing amino acid strand and the new amino acid brought by the tRNA.

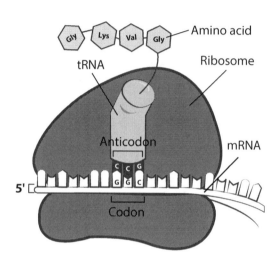

Figure 8.8. Translation

The translation process stops when a stop codon is reached in the sequence. These codons activate a protein called a release factor, which binds to the ribosome. The ribosome, which is made of two proteins, will split apart after the release factor binds. This releases the newly formed amino acid chain.

PRACTICE QUESTIONS

10. At an ACU codon, the amino acid threonine will be inserted in the polypeptide. Which of the following anticodons would be found on the tRNA molecule that carries threonine?

   A) ACU

   B) UCA

   C) TGA

   D) UGA

11. Which of the following causes translation to end?

   A) Anticodons bind to the ribosome.

   B) Stop codons are reached by the ribosome.

C) Codons are misread by the ribosomes.

D) tRNA binds to release factor.

Mutations

The DNA sequence can sometimes undergo a **mutation**, which is a change in the base-pair sequence of the DNA strand. A mutation can be benign, or silent, meaning it has no effect, or it can cause a change in the protein structure.

One way a gene can be changed permanently is through a **point mutation**, where a single base in the sequence of a gene changes. This can happen through a single base substitution, insertion, or deletion. If one base (or a few bases) in the sequence changes, this is called a **base substitution**. An **insertion** occurs when one base (or a few bases) is added to the sequence, and a deletion occurs when one nucleotide (or a few nucleotides) is lost from the sequence.

Adding or removing nucleotides from a stretch of DNA changes the total amount of DNA, which can influence how the gene is read by RNA polymerase and, ultimately, by ribosomes. This type of mutation is called a **frameshift mutation**. Occasionally, two breaks may occur in a chromosome, and the fragment that breaks away flips around and reattaches. This type of mutation is called a **chromosome inversion**.

Many mutations will not result in any change in the protein sequence at all. For example, if the sequence CCG mutated to CCA, there would be no change, because the codon produced by both sequences corresponds to the amino acid glycine.

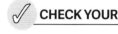

CHECK YOUR UNDERSTANDING

How would the consequences of a mutation in a gamete cell be different from those resulting from a mutation in a somatic cell?

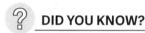

DID YOU KNOW?

Sickle cell anemia is caused by a point mutation. A single change in the base-pair sequence from a T to an A changes a codon from GAA to GUA, which changes the amino acid from glutamate to valine. The resulting hemoglobin protein is elongated and cannot carry oxygen as effectively.

PRACTICE QUESTIONS

12. Tay-Sachs disease is caused by a four-codon insertion that causes errors in the production of the enzyme beta-hexosaminidase. What kind of mutation causes Tay-Sachs disease?

A) point mutation

B) base substitution

C) frameshift mutation

D) deletion

13. A strand of DNA includes the nucleotide sequence ATGCTGG, but after replication the new strand has the sequence ATGCCTGG. What type of mutation occurred during replication?

A) insertion

B) deletion

C) frameshift mutation

D) chromosome inversion

Gene Regulation

In prokaryotes (e.g., bacteria) and some eukaryotes, genes are grouped together into a set of genes called an **operon**. The operon includes three parts:

- The **promoter** is the binding site for RNA polymerase and initiates transcription.
- The **operator** is the site to which an enzyme can bind to regulate transcription.
- The protein coding sequence includes the nucleotides that encode the protein.

Either negative or positive regulation is used to control the operon. In **negative regulation**, a gene will be expressed unless a repressor becomes attached. In **positive regulation**, genes are expressed only when an activator attaches to initiate expression.

The expression of DNA can also be controlled by changes to the structure of DNA. Tightening how tightly bound the chromatin is in the nucleus will restrict access to the DNA. Modifications to histone proteins can also inhibit or allow access to DNA..

PRACTICE QUESTION

14. Which of the following is necessary to initiate the transcription of a gene?
  A) DNA polymerase
  B) promoter
  C) centromere
  D) tRNA

Genetics

Genotype

Genetics is the study of genes and how they are passed down to offspring. Before the discovery of genes, there were many theories about how traits are passed to offspring. One of the dominant theories in the nineteenth century was blending inheritance, which stated that the genetic material from the parents would mix to form that of the children in the same way that two colors might mix.

The idea was eventually displaced by the current theory, which is based on the concept of a **gene**, which is a region of DNA that codes for a specific protein. Multiple versions of the same gene, called **alleles**, account for variation in a population.

During sexual reproduction, offspring receive a single copy of every gene from each parent. These two genes may be identical, making the individual **homozygous**, or they may be different, making the individual **heterozygous** for that gene. In a heterozygous individual, the genes do not blend; instead they act separately, with one often being completely or partially suppressed.

An organism's **genotype** is its complete genetic code. **Phenotype** is an organism's observable characteristics, such as height, eye color, skin color, and hair color. Although the genotype of two people might be different, each person could have the same phenotype, depending on which alleles are dominant or recessive. For example, the two types of roses Rr and RR are both red, meaning they have the same phenotype. However, they have a different genotype, with one rose type being heterozygous and the other being homozygous.

Two organisms with the same genotype may also have different phenotypes. The same genotype may be expressed differently based on environmental factors or the presence of other genes (a process called **epistasis**). For example, two plants with the same genotype may grow to different heights depending on the amount of sunlight available.

PRACTICE QUESTION

15. An individual's phenotype is the

    A) number of genes encoded by their DNA.

    B) physical traits encoded in their DNA.

    C) physical features determined by ribosomes.

    D) number of their traits repressed by modification.

 HELPFUL HINT

Natural selection acts on an organism's phenotype, not its genotype. Only alleles that affect an organism's fitness will be selected for or against.

Mendel's Laws

The idea that individual genes are passed down from parents to their children was conceived by **Gregor Mendel**. Mendel used various plants to test his ideas, but his best-known work is with pea plants. During the course of his work, he discovered that the plants had heritable features, meaning features that were passed from parent to offspring.

Mendel came up with three laws to describe genetic inheritance: the law of segregation, the law of independent assortment, and the law of dominance. The **law of segregation** states that genes come in allele pairs (if the organism is diploid, which most are) and that each parent can pass only a single allele down to its child. Thus, each individual has a pair of alleles for each gene: one from the father and one from the mother (in sexual reproduction). The law of segregation also states that the alleles must separate during meiosis so that only one is given to each gamete.

The **law of independent assortment** states that genes responsible for different traits are passed on independently. Thus, there is not necessarily a correlation between two genes. For example, if a mother is tall and has brown hair, she might pass on her genes for tallness to her child, but perhaps not the ones for brown hair.

Lastly, the **law of dominance** states that some alleles are dominant and some are recessive. **Dominant alleles** will mask the behavior of recessive ones. For example, red might be dominant in a rose, and white might be recessive. Thus, if a homozygous red rose mates with a homozygous white rose, all of their offspring will be red. Although the white gene allele will be present, it will not be expressed.

When writing the genetic information for a genotype, the dominant allele is written as a capital letter (A), while the recessive is written as a lowercase (a). A homozygous genotype can be AA or aa, and a heterozygous genotype will be Aa.

16. What does Mendel's law of segregation state?

A) Genes responsible for different traits are inherited independently.

B) Each parent passes one allele to each offspring.

C) Heritable features are passed on from parent to offspring.

D) The dominant allele is inherited more often than the recessive allele.

Monohybrid and Dihybrid Crosses

A **genetic cross** is a method in genetic experimentation in which a scientist intentionally breeds two individual parent organisms in order to produce an offspring that carries genetic material from both parents. The pair of parents is called the parental generation, or **P generation**. The offspring of this initial breeding is known as the first filial generation, or **F1 generation**. If the F1 generation is intentionally bred as well, the offspring of this generation is known as the second filial generation, or **F2 generation**. This pattern of naming continues on as more generations are bred during experimentation.

> **HELPFUL HINT**
>
> If an organism is described as true-breeding for a specific trait, it is homozygous for that trait and will pass it on to its offspring.

The purpose of these genetic crosses is to isolate and study traits as they are passed through the generations. In **monohybrid** crosses, the P generation is selected based on one particular trait—one parent possesses the dominant trait, while the other possesses the recessive trait. For example, in one of his pea experiments, Mendel selectively bred one plant with the dominant yellow seed trait with another plant that had the recessive green seed trait. The parent with the dominant trait can have a genotype that is either homozygous (YY) or heterozygous (Yy), while the parent with the recessive trait has a homozygous genotype (yy).

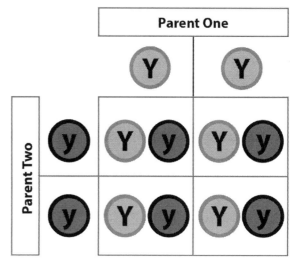

Figure 8.9. Punnett Square: Monohybrid Cross of Seed Color

The phenotype of the resulting F1 generation can be predicted using a **Punnett square**. This diagram determines the probability that an offspring will inherit a particular genotype. For monohybrid crosses, the Punnett square has only four possible combinations for a genotype, each with a 25 percent chance of occurring.

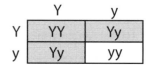

Figure 8.10. Punnett Square: Monohybrid Cross of Seed Color

The probability that a certain genotype combination will occur is the Punnett ratio. For example, if two heterozygous yellow pea plants (Yy) are crossed, the Punnett square shows that there is a 3/4 probability that the offspring will be yellow and a 1/4 probability the offspring will be green. Therefore, this mono-hybrid cross has a Punnett ratio of 3:1.

In a **dihybrid cross**, the P generation is selected for two traits that differ between the two parents. One of Mendel's pea experiments included the dihybrid cross of a P generation that bred one parent with the two dominant traits (yellow and round) with a parent that had two recessive traits (green and wrinkled). The resulting Punnett square displays sixteen possible combinations of genotypes for these two traits. The Punnett ratio for this is 9:3:3:1 because there is a:

- 9/16 probability that the offspring will be yellow and smooth
- 3/16 probability that the offspring will be yellow and wrinkled
- 3/16 probability that the offspring will be green and smooth
- 1/16 probability that the offspring will be green and wrinkled

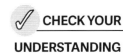

CHECK YOUR UNDERSTANDING

If the parent with the dominant yellow seed trait has a homozygous trait of YY, then there is a 100 percent chance that the F1 generation will express the yellow seed trait. How does this change if the YY parent instead has a Yy genotype?

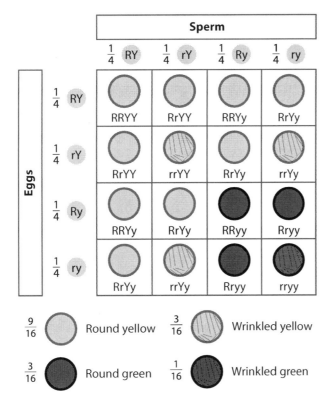

Figure 8.11. Punnett Square: Dihybrid Cross of Seed Color and Shape

PRACTICE QUESTIONS

17. The height of a certain plant is determined by a gene with two alleles—tall and short. Tallness is a recessive trait. If a homozygous tall plant is crossed with a homozygous short plant, what percentage of the F2 generation will be tall?

    A) 0 percent
    B) 25 percent
    C) 50 percent
    D) 100 percent

18. In a certain plant, having the dominant allele R results in bright-red seeds, and the recessive allele r results in pale-pink seeds. In the first generation, a scientist crosses a true-breeding RR plant with a recessive rr plant. The F1 plant is then crossed with itself, resulting in the F2 generation. In the F2 generation, what percentage of the plants will have bright red seeds?

A) 25 percent

B) 50 percent

C) 75 percent

D) 100 percent

Non-Mendelian Genetics

Mendel's laws apply to traits that are controlled by only one gene that has two possible alleles with a dominant/recessive relationship. Many traits do not fit these qualifications and will show inheritance patterns that are different from what Mendelian genetics would predict.

Gene linkage occurs with genes that are situated close together on a chromosome and thus are more likely to be inherited together. Tracking the frequency of linked genes being transmitted together can help researchers determine the physical relationship between genes. All genes have a 50 percent chance of being inherited with any other gene. Genes that are paired with another gene more than 50 percent of the time are more likely to be linked; the higher the percentage, the closer the genes are in distance to one another.

Sex-linked genes are located on the **sex chromosome** of each individual. All females have two **X chromosomes**, while all males have both an **X** and a **Y chromosome**. Genes that are located on the Y chromosome result in traits that are expressed only in the males of a species. Because females have two X chromosomes (and thus carry two alleles), the dominant allele will express itself for X-linked traits. Males, however, have only one allele for every X gene. As a result, the trait will be expressed whether it is dominant or recessive.

Non-Mendelian inheritance patterns can also be seen when alleles do not have a binary dominant/recessive relationship. The appearance of two dominant alleles creates an effect called **codominance**, in which both dominant genes are expressed in the individual. This effect is responsible for the human blood type AB, as the gene for blood types A and B are both dominant. **Incomplete dominance** occurs when one allele is not completely dominant over the other. For example, if the flower color red is incompletely dominant over the color white, offspring with both alleles will have pink flowers (a blend of red and white).

 DID YOU KNOW?

Color blindness and hemophilia are both X-linked disorders: they are carried by females but appear more frequently in males.

PRACTICE QUESTIONS

19. Which of the following statements describes the expression of X-linked traits?

A) X-linked traits are expressed more often in men.

B) X-linked traits are expressed more often in women.

C) X-linked traits are expressed equally in men and women.

D) X-linked traits are expressed only in men who carry the dominant allele.

20. When a scientist crosses a red flower with a white flower, the F1 generation has pink flowers. In this flower, the allele for red is

   A) dominant over white.

   B) codominant with white.

   C) incompletely dominant over white.

   D) recessive to white.

Introduction of Genetic Variation

Sexual reproduction introduces genetic variation into each generation. During meiosis, the **independent assortment** of chromosomes gives each gamete a unique subset of genes from the parent. When a gamete combines with another to form a zygote, the result is a genetically unique organism that has a different gene composition from either of the parents.

The process of meiosis also introduces genetic variation during **crossing-over**, which occurs in prophase I when homologous chromosomes pair along their lengths. Each gene on each chromosome becomes aligned with its sister gene. When crossing-over occurs, a DNA sequence is broken and crisscrossed, creating a new chromatid with pieces of each of the original homologous chromosomes.

Random fertilization, the random pairing of sperm and egg, also produces genetic variation. Organisms produce millions of gametes, so no matter how many times a pair breeds, it is next to impossible to get two children that have the same genotype (except identical twins).

PRACTICE QUESTION

21. Which of the following is NOT a way that meiosis increases genetic variation?

   A) creating haploid sex cells that will be randomly fertilized

   B) allowing for the exchange of genetic material between chromosomes

   C) increasing the probability of mutations in the nucleotide sequence of DNA

   D) sorting each set of homologous chromosomes independently

The Cell

The **cell** is the smallest unit of life that can reproduce on its own. All higher organisms are composed of cells, which are specialized to perform the many processes that keep organisms alive and allow them to reproduce.

Parts of the Cell

Although the cell is the smallest unit of life, there are many small bodies, called **organelles**, which exist within it. These organelles are required for the many processes that take place inside a cell.

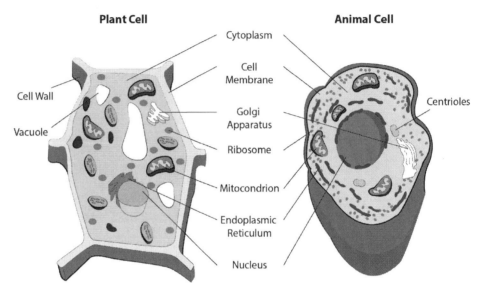

Figure 8.12. Plant and Animal Cell Organelles

- The **mitochondria** are the organelles responsible for making ATP within the cell. Mitochondria have several layers of membranes used to assist the electron transport chain. This pathway uses energy provided by molecules, such as glucose or fat (lipid), to generate ATP through the transfer of electrons.

- A **vacuole** is a small body used to transfer materials within and out of the cell. It has a membrane of its own and can carry things such as cell waste, sugars, or proteins.

- The **nucleus** of a eukaryotic cell contains all of its genetic information in the form of DNA. In the nucleus, DNA replication and transcription occur. In the eukaryotic cell, after transcription, the mRNA is exported out of the nucleus into the cytosol for use.

- The **endoplasmic reticulum** (ER) is used for translating mRNA into proteins and transporting proteins out of the cell. The rough endoplasmic reticulum has many ribosomes attached to it, which function as the cell's machinery in transforming RNA into protein. The smooth endoplasmic reticulum is associated with the production of fats and steroid hormones.

- A **ribosome** is a small two-protein unit that reads mRNA and, with the assistance of transport proteins, creates an amino acid.
- The **Golgi apparatus** collects, packages, and distributes the proteins produced by ribosomes.
- **Chloroplasts** are plant organelles where the reactions of photosynthesis take place.

PRACTICE QUESTIONS

22. Muscle tissues often require quick bursts of energy. As a result, which of the following organelles would most likely be found in higher than normal amounts in muscle cells?

A) ribosomes

B) chloroplasts

C) vacuoles

D) mitochondria

23. Which of the following is found in plant cells but not in animal cells?

A) cell wall

B) Golgi apparatus

C) plasma membrane

D) proteins

Cell Membrane

The **cell membrane** surrounds the cell and controls what enters and leaves. It is composed of compounds called **phospholipids** that consist of an alkane tail and a phospho-group head. The alkane lipid tail is hydrophobic, meaning it will not allow water to pass through. The phosphate group head is hydrophilic—it will allow water to pass through. The arrangement of these molecules forms a bilayer, which has a hydrophobic middle layer. In this manner, the cell is able to control the import and export of various substances into the cell.

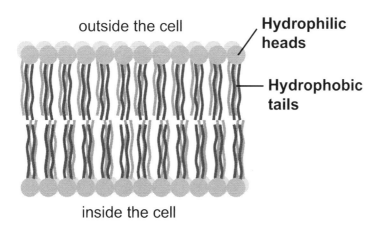

Figure 8.13. Cell Membrane Bilayer

In addition to the phospholipid bilayer, the cell membrane often includes proteins, which perform a variety of functions. Some proteins are used as receptors, which allow the cell to interact with its surroundings. Others are **transmembrane proteins**, meaning they cross the entire membrane. These types of proteins are usually channels that allow the transportation of molecules into and out of the cell.

There are two major types of transportation that cells use to move substances across the cell membrane: active transport and passive transport.

Passive transport does not require energy and allows molecules, such as water, to passively diffuse across the cell membrane. **Facilitated diffusion** is a form of passive transport that does not require energy but does require the use of proteins located on the cell membrane. These transport proteins typically have a "channel" running through the core of a protein that is specific to a certain type of molecule. For example, a transport protein for sodium only allows sodium to flow through the channel.

Active transport requires energy and can perform two basic tasks:

1. move a molecule against the concentration gradient (from low concentration to high)

2. import or export a bulky molecule, such as a sugar or a protein, across the cell membrane.

Active transport requires the use of proteins and energy in the form of ATP. The ATP produced by the cell binds to the proteins in the cell membrane and is hydrolyzed, producing the energy required to change the conformational structure of the protein. This change in the structure of the protein allows the protein to funnel molecules across the cell membrane.

PRACTICE QUESTIONS

24. Which of the following cellular processes does NOT use ATP?

A) facilitated diffusion

B) DNA replication

C) active transport through the cell membrane

D) movement of the Mot complex in a flagellum

25. Which of the following is NOT one of the functions of proteins found in the phospholipid bilayer of a cell membrane?

A) to break down material that enters through the cell membrane

B) to act as receptors that recognize and transmit hormonal messages

C) to provide an attachment point for other cells

D) to transport material across the membrane into the cell

Tonicity

The balance of water in the cell is one of its most important regulatory mechanisms. Water enters or exits the cell through a process called **osmosis**. This movement of water does not usually require energy. The movement is regulated by a **tonicity**, the concentration of solutes in the cell. Solutes can be salt ions, such as sodium or chlorine, or other molecules, such as sugar, amino acids, or proteins.

The difference in tonicity between the cell and its outside environment governs the transportation of water into and out of the cell. For example, if there is a higher tonicity inside the cell, then water will enter the cell. If there is a higher tonicity outside the cell, the water will leave the cell. This is due to a driving force called the **chemiosmotic potential**, which attempts to make tonicity equal across a membrane.

There are three terms used to describe a cell's tonicity:

- When a cell is in an **isotonic** environment, the same concentration of solutes exists inside and outside the cell. There will be no transport of water in this case.

- When a cell is in a **hypertonic** environment, the concentration of solutes outside the cell is higher than that inside the cell. The cell will lose water to the environment and shrivel. This is what happens if a cell is placed into a salty solution.

- When a cell is in a **hypotonic** environment, the concentration of solutes outside the cell is lower than that inside the cell. The cell will absorb water from the environment and swell, becoming turgid.

 HELPFUL HINT

Salting meats creates a hypertonic environment that dehydrates microbes, including disease-causing bacteria. In this hypertonic environment, bacterial cells lose so much water they can no longer function, which protects the meat from infection.

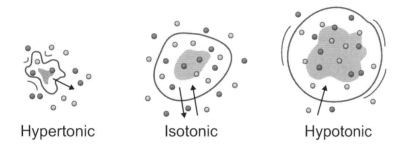

Hypertonic   Isotonic   Hypotonic

Figure 8.14. Tonicity

PRACTICE QUESTION

26. A student places a cell with a 50 mM intracellular ion content into a solution containing a 20 mM ion content. Which of the following will happen in this system?

   A) Water will move out of the cell, decreasing the size of the cell.

   B) Water will move into the cell, increasing the size of the cell.

   C) Ions will move into the cell.

   D) There will be no movement of water or ions across the cell membrane.

Mitosis and Meiosis

The cell cycle is the process cells go through as they live, grow, and divide to produce new cells. The cell cycle can be divided into four primary phases:

1. G1 phase: growth phase one
2. S phase: DNA replication
3. G2 phase: growth phase two
4. Mitotic phase: The cell undergoes mitosis and splits into two cells.

Together, the G1, S, and G2 phases are known as **interphase**. During these phases, which usually take up 80 to 90 percent of the total time in a cell cycle, the cell is growing and conducting normal cell functions.

The process of cell division is called **mitosis**. When a cell divides, it needs to make sure that each copy of the cell has a roughly equal amount of the necessary elements, including DNA, proteins, and organelles. In multicellular organisms, mitosis occurs in somatic (body) cells that contain a pair of homologous chromosomes. The two resulting daughter cells will have identical genetic material.

The mitotic phase is separated into five substages:

- **Prophase**: In prophase, the DNA in the cell winds into chromatin, and each pair of duplicated chromosomes becomes joined. The mitotic spindle, which later pulls apart the chromosomes, forms and drifts to each end of the cell.

- **Prometaphase**: In this phase, the nuclear membrane, which holds the DNA, dissolves, allowing the chromosomes to come free. The chromosomes now start to attach to microtubules linked to the centrioles.

- **Metaphase**: The centrioles, with microtubules attached to the chromosomes, are now on opposite sides of the cell. The chromosomes align in the middle of the cell, and the microtubules begin contracting.

- **Anaphase**: In anaphase, the chromosomes move to separate sides of the cell, and the cell structure begins to lengthen, pulling apart as it goes.

- **Telophase and Cytokinesis**: In this last part of the cell cycle, the cell membrane splits, and two new daughter cells are formed. The nucleolus, containing the DNA, re-forms.

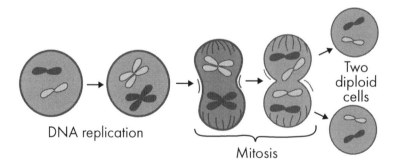

Figure 8.15. Mitosis

Meiosis is cellular division that creates gametes (sex cells). The dividing cell starts with a set of homologous chromosomes (*2n*), but the four resulting

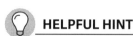

HELPFUL HINT

The Cell Cycle

Go Donna Go, Make Children!

Growth phase 1

DNA Synthesis

Growth phase 2

Mitosis

Cytokinesis

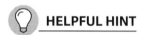

HELPFUL HINT

Mitosis

I Passed My Anatomy Test

Interphase

Prophase

Metaphase

Anaphase

Telophase

daughter cells will each have only one set of chromosomes (1*n*). There are two consecutive stages of meiosis known as meiosis I and meiosis II. These two stages are further broken down into four stages each.

Meiosis I

1. Prophase I: The chromosomes condense, using histone proteins, and become paired. Microtubules attach to the chromosomes and centrioles and begin to align them in the middle of the cell.

2. Metaphase I: The chromosomes align in the middle of the cell and begin to pull apart from one another.

3. Anaphase I: The homologous chromosomes separate and move toward opposite sides of the cell.

4. Telophase I: The cells separate, and each cell now has one copy each of a homologous chromosome.

Meiosis II

1. Prophase II: A spindle forms and aligns the chromosomes; no crossing-over occurs.

2. Metaphase II: The chromosomes again align at the metaphase plate.

3. Anaphase II: The sister chromatids pull apart to opposite ends of the cell.

4. Telophase II: The cell splits apart, resulting in four unique daughter cells.

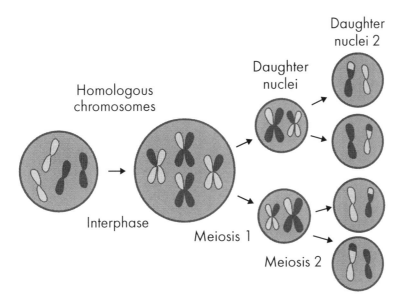

Figure 8.16. Meiosis

PRACTICE QUESTIONS

27. A scientist takes DNA samples from a cell culture at two different times, with each sample having the same cell count. In the first sample, he finds that there is 6.5 pg of DNA, whereas in the second sample, he finds that there is 13 pg of DNA. In which stage of the cell cycle is the first sample?

A) interphase G1

B) interphase S

C) interphase G2

D) mitotic phase

28. At the end of which phase of mitosis are chromosomes first clearly visible under a light microscope?

A) interphase

B) prophase

C) metaphase

D) anaphase

Microorganisms and Infectious Disease

When an organism establishes an opportunistic relationship with a host, the process is called **infection**. There are four stages of the infection process. Infections can be mild or severe, and the acuteness of an infection depends on the disease-causing potential of the infectious agent and the ability of the body to defend itself. Infections can be caused by many different infectious agents.

- **Bacteria** are single-celled prokaryotic organisms that are responsible for many common infections, such as strep throat, urinary tract infections, and many food-borne illnesses.

- **Viruses** are composed of a nucleic acid (DNA or RNA) wrapped in a protein capsid. They invade host cells and hijack cell machinery to reproduce. Viral infections include the common cold, influenza, and human immunodeficiency virus (HIV).

- **Protozoa** are single-celled eukaryotic organisms. Protozoan infections include giardia (an intestinal infection) and sleeping sickness (trypanosomiasis).

- **Fungi** are a group of eukaryotic organisms that include yeasts, molds, and mushrooms. Common fungal infections are athlete's foot, ringworm, and oral and vaginal yeast infections.

Parasitic diseases are caused by **parasites** that live in or on the human body and use its resources. Common human parasites include worms (tapeworms, for example), flukes, and ectoparasites, such as lice and ticks, which live on the outside of the body.

Infections travel from person to person via the **chain of infection**. The chain starts with a causative organism, such as a bacteria or virus. The organism needs a **reservoir**, or place to live. This may be biological, such as people or animals, or environmental. For example, in a medical office, equipment and office surfaces

HELPFUL HINT

Infectious disease precautions are categorized based on how the disease is transmitted. For example, droplet precautions require only a surgical mask, but airborne precautions require an N-95 respirator to prevent transmission.

may act as reservoirs. In order to spread, the infectious agent needs a way to **exit** the reservoir, such as being expelled as droplets during a sneeze.

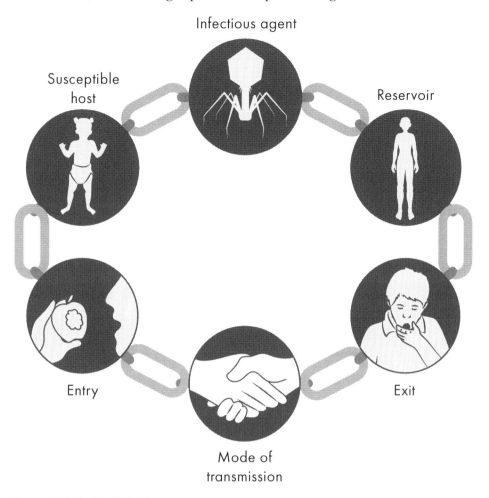

Figure 8.17. Chain of Infection

For the infection chain to continue, the infectious agent needs to encounter a susceptible **host**—a person who can become infected. Finally, the infectious agent needs a way to enter the host, such as through inhalation or drinking contaminated water. There are a variety of **modes of transmission** for infectious agents.

- **Direct contact** is transmission from one infected person to another during physical contact with blood or other body fluids (the transmission of herpes during sexual intercourse, for example).

- **Indirect contact** is transmission of the disease through a nonbiological reservoir (drinking water contaminated with giardia, for example).

- **Droplets** are infectious agents trapped in moisture that are expelled when an infected person sneezes or coughs. They can enter the respiratory system of other people and cause infection (for example, the transmission of influenza when an infected person sneezes).

- Some droplets are light enough to remain airborne, meaning people may inhale infectious agents from the air long after the initial cough or sneeze (measles, for example, which can live in **airborne droplets** for up to two hours).

- Some diseases are carried by organisms called **vectors** that spread the disease; the infection does not require direct physical contact between people (mosquitoes carrying malaria, for example).

PRACTICE QUESTIONS

29. The common cold, influenza, and HIV are caused by which type of infectious agent?

    A) bacteria

    B) protozoan

    C) virus

    D) fungus

30. How are vector-borne diseases transmitted?

    A) Fluids are transferred during direct contact.

    B) Small droplets are inhaled.

    C) Contaminated water is consumed.

    D) Organisms carry the infectious agent.

Answer Key

1. **A)** Organic compounds must contain carbon. They may contain other elements, including phosphorous, nitrogen, or oxygen.

2. **D)** Guanine is a nucleic acid, not a polysaccharide.

3. **A)** Most lipids have a polar head made of phosphate or glycerol.

4. **D)** A monomer is a building block used to build large molecules such as proteins. Amino acids are the monomers used to build proteins.

5. **B)** Uracil is a nucleotide found in RNA, not DNA.

6. **B)** This sequence correctly matches each nucleotide, has the correct orientation, and does not contain the nucleotide uracil (which is found in RNA).

7. **A)** DNA is organized into chromosomes using histone proteins. First, DNA is wound into nucleosomes by histones. Next, the nucleosomes are wound into chromatin, which is wound even tighter to form chromosomes.

8. **B)** DNA polymerase cannot replicate the end of a DNA strand, so that section of the DNA is lost during replication.

9. **C)** DNA ligase joins broken strands of DNA. Enzymes are often named for their function: *ligate* means "to join or tie together."

10. **D)** Anticodons and codons are complementary: the complement of the codon ACU is the anticodon UGA.

11. **B)** Translation will end when the ribosome encounters a stop codon. The stop codons activate a protein called release factor, which will bind to the ribosome and release the protein.

12. **C)** In a frameshift mutation, insertions of nucleotides in numbers other than three will shift all the following codons read by the tRNA, producing a dysfunctional protein.

13. **A)** This is an example of an insertion mutation. A cytosine has been inserted into the sequence in the mutated sequence.

14. **B)** A promoter is necessary to initiate gene transcription. If a promoter is not present, the gene cannot be expressed.

15. **B)** Phenotype is how genotype is expressed as physical features.

16. **B)** The law of segregation states that each parent passes one allele to each offspring.

17. **A)** All the offspring will have one copy of each allele, so they will be short because that is the dominant trait.

	T	T
t	Tt	Tt
t	Tt	Tt

18. **C)** Use Punnett squares to find the result of each cross. The F1 generation will all have the genotype Rr:

F1	R	R
r	Rr	Rr
r	Rr	Rr

In the F2 generation, 75 percent of the plants will carry the dominant R allele:

F2	R	r
R	RR	Rr
r	Rr	rr

19. **A)** X-linked traits are expressed more often in men because they carry only one copy of the gene and so will express the gene whether the allele is dominant or recessive.

20. **C)** When incomplete dominance occurs, neither allele is dominant, and the offspring will have a phenotype that is a blend of the two alleles.

21. **C)** Meiosis does not increase the probability of mutations. Mutations are caused by environmental factors (such as radiation) or mistakes in DNA replication.

22. **D)** The mitochondria found in cells are what power the cell and provide it with the energy it needs to carry out its life functions. Muscle cells need a lot of ATP in order to provide the energy needed for movement and exercise.

23. **A)** Both plant and animal cells have carbohydrates, nucleic acids, proteins, and lipids. Plants and animals have similar organelles, including the Golgi apparatus; however, plant cells have a cell wall and animal cells do not.

24. **A)** Facilitated diffusion is a form of passive transport across the cell membrane and does not use energy.

25. **A)** Cytoplasm breaks down material that enters through the cell membrane.

26. **B)** The concentration of ions is higher inside the cell than outside, so water will move into the cell from the environment, increasing the size of the cell.

27. **A)** During interphase G1, the cell has not replicated its DNA. During the other three phases listed, the cell would have replicated its DNA, doubling the amount of DNA in the cell.

28. **B)** During prophase, the DNA replicated during interphase condenses into chromosomes, which are clearly visible under a light microscope.

29. **C)** Viruses are responsible for the common cold, influenza, and HIV (human immunodeficiency virus).

30. **D)** Vector-borne diseases are carried by other organisms (called vectors) between hosts.

9 | Chemistry

The Structure of the Atom

The **atom** is the basic building block of all physical matter. It is composed of three subatomic particles: protons, electrons, and neutrons. A **proton** is a positively charged subatomic particle with a mass of approximately 1.007 atomic mass units. The number of protons in an atom determines which **element** it is. For example, an atom with one proton is hydrogen, and an atom with twelve protons is carbon.

A **neutron** is a non-charged subatomic particle with a mass of approximately 1.008 atomic mass units. The number of neutrons in an atom does not affect its chemical properties but will influence its rate of radioactivity. Both protons and neutrons are found in the center, or **nucleus**, of the atom.

Lastly, an **electron** is a negatively charged subatomic particle with a mass of approximately 0.00055 atomic mass units.

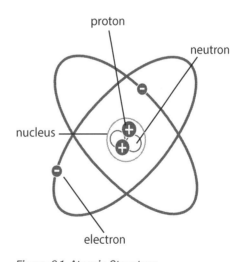

Figure 9.1. Atomic Structure

The number of electrons and protons in an atom determines its charge. An atom with more protons than electrons is a positive **cation**, and an atom with more electrons than protons is a negative **anion**. Cations and anions are collectively referred to as **ions**.

The modern concept of the atom, which provided the basis for all of chemistry, was first laid out in John Dalton's **Atomic Theory**, which was developed in 1808. Atomic theory states the following:

1. An element is composed of atoms, which are extremely small, indivisible particles. Although we now know that atoms are composed of smaller units such as protons, electrons, and neutrons, it is still recognized that atoms are the basic building blocks of matter.

2. Each individual element has a set of properties that are distinct and different from that of other elements.

3. Atoms cannot be created, destroyed, or transformed through physical changes. We now know that atoms can be created or destroyed, although this requires a massive amount of energy. Furthermore, radioactive elements can be transformed into other elements.

4. Compounds are defined by a specific ratio of atoms that are combined with one another, and the relative numbers and types of atoms are constant in any given compound.

PRACTICE QUESTIONS

1. Which of the following subatomic particles are found in the nucleus of an atom?

    A) protons only

    B) electrons only

    C) protons and neutrons only

    D) protons, electrons, and neutrons

2. What is the charge of an atom with five protons and seven electrons?

    A) 12

    B) −12

    C) 2

    D) −2

Electron Configuration

The atom consists of a nucleus of protons and neutrons surrounded by orbiting electrons. The nucleus is very dense and contains the majority of mass in the atom. The actual size of the atom, due to the large orbits of the electrons, is much larger than the nucleus.

Electron configuration refers to the location of an atom's electrons. Electrons surround the nucleus in clouds called **orbitals**, each of which holds two electrons. These orbitals are grouped into **subshells**, each of which has a particular shape and holds a specific number of electrons. There are four orbital shapes:

- s has 1 orbital and holds $1 \times 2 = 2$ electrons
- p has 3 orbitals and holds $3 \times 2 = 6$ electrons
- d has 5 orbitals and holds $5 \times 2 = 10$ electrons
- f has 7 orbitals and holds $7 \times 2 = 14$ electrons

Subshells are grouped into **shells** identified by integers (1, 2, 3, …). Shells with smaller integers are smaller and are located close to the nucleus; shells with larger numbers are larger and are located farther from the nucleus.

The location of an electron can be described by its shell number and subshell letter. For example, the single electron in hydrogen is in orbital $1s$. The number of electrons in each orbital is written as a superscript, so the full electron configuration for hydrogen is $1s^1$. The notation for the first four shells is shown in Table 9.1.

TABLE 9.1. Electron Configuration Notation				
SHELL	**SUBSHELL**	**NO. OF ORBITALS**	**NO. OF ELECTRONS IN SUBSHELL**	**NOTATION FOR FULL SUBSHELL**
1	s	1	2	$1s^2$
2	s	1	2	$2s^2$
	p	3	6	$2p^6$
3	s	1	2	$3s^2$
	p	3	6	$3p^6$
	d	5	10	$3d^{10}$
4	s	1	2	$4s^2$
	p	3	6	$4p^6$
	d	5	10	$4d^{10}$
	f	7	14	$4f^{14}$

Electrons fill orbitals in a specific order, starting with low-energy orbitals and then filling in higher-energy orbitals. The general order in which electrons are filled is shown in Figure 9.2. Note that not all elements follow this order: large elements that have electrons in d and f orbitals will often fill orbitals in unpredictable ways.

The reactivity of each individual atom is determined by the number of electrons in its outermost, or **valence**, shell. Typically, the closer an atom is to reaching a full valence shell, the more reactive it is. Elements that have a single electron in a shell (such as sodium: last orbital $3s^1$) or that need only a single electron to fill a shell (such as chlorine: last orbital $3p^5$) are the most reactive.

There are some elements that are not reactive at all. These are the noble gases, which possess a full valence shell. Thus, they

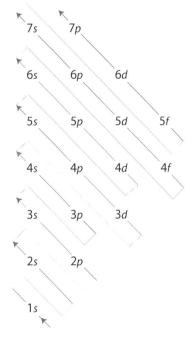

increasing energy

1s 2s 2p 3s 3p 4s 3d 4p 5s 4d 5p 6s …

Figure 9.2. Filling Electron Orbitals

have no free electrons with which to react. In chemistry, there are no common reactions that occur with a noble gas.

PRACTICE QUESTIONS

3. Which of the following is the electron configuration for phosphorus?

A) $1s^2 2s^2 2p^6 3s^2 3p^3$

B) $1s^2 2s^2 2p^6 3s^2 3p^6$

C) $1s^2 2p^6 3s^2 3p^3$

D) $1s^2 2s^2 2p^2 3s^2 3p^3 4s^2 4p^3$

4. How many electrons are needed to complete the valence shell of the noble gases?

A) 0

B) 1

C) 2

D) 3

The Periodic Table of the Elements

Reading the Periodic Table

The **periodic table** is a table used to organize and characterize the various elements. The table was first proposed by Dmitri Mendeleev in 1869, and a similar organization system is still used today. In the table, each column is called a **group**, and each row is called a **period**. Elements in the same column have similar electron configurations and the same number of electrons in their valence shells.

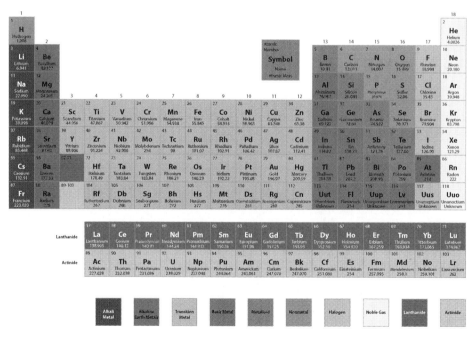

Figure 9.3. The Periodic Table of the Elements

Each cell in the table includes the symbol for the element, which is a letter or set of letters; for example, C for carbon and Fe for iron. The number at the top of each cell in the table is the **atomic number**. This represents the number of protons in the element. The number below the element symbol is the **atomic mass**, which represents the total mass of the element (atomic mass – atomic number = # of neutrons).

Figure 9.4. Reading the Periodic Table

Because atoms of the same element can have different numbers of neutrons, elements have no single standard atomic mass. Instead, the atomic mass is the weighted average of all commonly found species of the element. For this reason, it is almost never a whole number. For example, a small amount of carbon actually has an atomic mass of 13, possessing seven neutrons instead of the usual six, giving carbon an atomic mass of 12.011. Atoms of the same element with different numbers of neutrons are called **isotopes**.

PRACTICE QUESTIONS

5. The number of neutrons in an atom is equal to

    A) the atomic mass minus the number of electrons.

    B) the number of protons plus the number of electrons.

    C) the number of protons minus the number of electrons.

    D) the atomic mass minus the atomic number.

6. Which elements have the same number of electrons in their valence shell? (Refer to the periodic table.)

    A) Na, K, Ca

    B) Mg, Be, Cr

    C) F, Cl, Br

    D) P, N, C

Groups of Elements

Below are the important properties of the groups in the periodic table of elements.

Group 1 (The Alkali Metals): The elements in group 1 are all silvery metals that are soft and can be easily crushed or cut. They all possess a single valence electron, meaning they easily form +1 cations and are highly reactive. Because these metals are so reactive, they are not usually found in their pure form but instead are found as ionic compounds.

Group 2 (The Alkali Earth Metals): The elements in group 2 are also silvery metals that are soft. These metals contain two valence electrons, so they are not as reactive as those in group 1. However, they are still highly reactive: they form +2 cations and are found in ionic compounds.

Groups 3 – 12 (The Transition Metals): The elements from groups 3 to 12 are the transition metals and are all capable of conducting electricity (some better than others). Because their valence electrons are in *d* orbitals, their electron configurations are complex, and they form many different compounds and bonds. Transition metals are moderately reactive and malleable and can conduct electricity due to the capability of gaining and losing many electrons in their outer electron shell.

Groups 13 and 14 (Semi-metallic): The elements in groups 13 and 14 are semi-metallic. They have moderate conductivity and are very soft. Elements in group 13 have three valence electrons, and elements in group 14 have four, allowing for five and four bonds, respectively.

Group 15: This group is characterized by a shift from the top of this group (gases) to the bottom (semi-metallic). This group has five valence electrons and can form three bonds. The semi-metallic elements, such as arsenic and antimony, can react in specific circumstances but are generally not considered reactive.

Group 16: This group is also characterized by a shift from gases at the top of the group to semi-metallic at the bottom. This group has six valence electrons and is quite reactive. The need to obtain only two more electrons to fill the valence shell means that these elements are electronegative and typically form an anion with a charge of −2. As a result, these elements are reactive and tend to bond with the alkali or alkali earth metals.

Group 17 (Halogens): The halogens are all gases, and all contain seven electrons in their valence shell. They are extremely reactive, much like the alkali metals. Due to their reactivity and gaseous form at room temperature, they are often hazardous to humans. Inhaling chlorine or fluorine, for example, is usually deadly. The halogens will react in order to obtain a single additional electron to fill their valence shell and typically have a charge of −1.

Group 18 (The Noble Gases): The noble gases have a full valence shell. Because their electron orbitals are already full, the noble gases are largely unreactive, except for a few rare exceptions. The heavier noble gases (xenon and radon) can sometimes react with other species under high temperature and pressure conditions.

PRACTICE QUESTIONS

7. Which of the following elements is an alkali metal?

   A) sodium

   B) oxygen

   C) neon

   D) iron

8. Which of the following elements will form an ion with a charge of −2? (Refer to the periodic table.)

   A) F and Be

   B) Cl and Br

C) Se and Br

D) Se and O

Trends in the Periodic Table

Some element properties can be predicted based on the placement of the element on the periodic table.

- **Atomic radius**, the distance from the center of the atom to its outermost electron shell, increases from right to left and top to bottom on the periodic table.

- **Electronegativity** measures how strongly an atom attracts electrons. In general, electronegativity increases from left to right and bottom to top on the periodic table with fluorine being the most electronegative element.

- **Ionization energy**, a measure of how much energy is required to remove an electron from an atom, increases from lower left to top right.

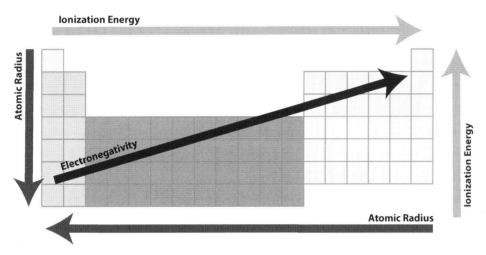

Figure 9.5. Trends in the Periodic Table

PRACTICE QUESTIONS

9. Which of the following elements is the most electronegative?

    A) radon (Rn)

    B) tin (Sn)

    C) sulfur (S)

    D) fluorine (F)

10. Which of the following elements has the smallest atomic radius?

    A) oxygen (O)

    B) boron (B)

    C) nitrogen (N)

    D) carbon (C)

Chemical Bonding

Atoms can exist on their own or bond together. When two or more atoms are held together by chemical bonds, they form a **molecule**. If the molecule contains more than one type of atom, it is a **compound**. Molecules and compounds form the smallest unit of a substance—for example, if water (H_2O) is broken down into hydrogen and oxygen atoms, it no longer has the unique properties of water. Molecules and compounds always have the same ratio of elements. Water, for example, always has two hydrogens for every one oxygen.

Intramolecular Forces

A chemical bond is a force that holds two atoms together. There are three primary types of bonds: ionic, covalent, and metallic.

In an **ionic bond**, one atom has lost electrons to the other, which results in a positive charge on one atom and a negative charge on the other atom. The bond is then a result of the electrostatic interaction between these positive and negative charges. For example, in the compound sodium chloride, sodium has lost an electron to chlorine, resulting in a positive charge on sodium and a negative charge on chlorine.

In a **covalent bond**, electrons are shared between two atoms; neither atom completely loses or gains an electron. This can be in the form of one pair of shared electrons (a single bond), two pairs (a double bond), or three pairs of electrons shared (triple bond). In diatomic oxygen gas, for example, the two oxygen molecules share two sets of electrons.

Covalent bonds are often depicted using Lewis diagrams, in which an electron is represented by a dot, and a shared pair of electrons is represented by a line.

Electrons within a covalent bond are not always shared equally. More electronegative atoms, which exert a strong pull on the electrons, will hold onto the electrons longer than less electronegative atoms. For example, oxygen is more electronegative than hydrogen, so in

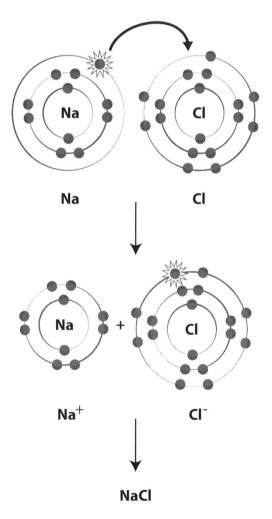

Figure 9.6. The Ionic Bond in Table Salt (NaCl)

H$_2$O (water), the oxygen has a slight negative charge, and both hydrogens have a slight positive charge. This imbalance is called **polarity**, and the small charge is called a **dipole**.

Water: H$_2$O

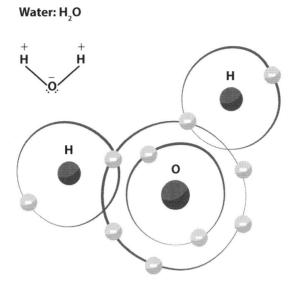

Figure 9.7. The Covalent Bond in Water (H$_2$O)

Note that there is a commonality between these two types of bonding. In both ionic and covalent bonding types, the bond results in each atom having a full valence shell of electrons. When bonding, atoms seek to find the most stable electron configuration. In the majority of cases, this means filling the valence shell of the atom either through the addition or removal of electrons.

Metallic bonds are created when metals form tightly packed arrays. Valence electrons are not attached to a particular atom and instead float freely among the positive metallic cations. This "sea" of electrons creates a strong bond that has high electrical and thermal conductivity.

 HELPFUL HINT

Water is often called the universal solvent because its strong dipole allows it to dissolve most polar and ionic compounds. Non-polar substances, such as oil, will not dissolve in water because they have no charge to interact with water's dipole.

PRACTICE QUESTIONS

11. Which of the following bonds is the most polar?

A) H—C

B) H—O

C) H—F

D) H—N

12. Which of the following elements is most likely to form an ionic bond?

A) argon

B) calcium

C) copper

D) nitrogen

Intermolecular Forces

What causes water to stick together, forming a liquid at room temperature but a solid at lower temperatures? Why do we need more heat and energy to increase the temperature of water compared to other substances? The answer is **intermolecular forces**: attractive or repulsive forces that occur between molecules. These are different from ionic and covalent bonds, which occur within a molecule.

The force of attraction between hydrogen and an extremely electronegative atom, such as oxygen or nitrogen, is known as a **hydrogen bond**. For example, in water (H_2O), oxygen atoms are attracted to the hydrogen atoms in nearby molecules, creating hydrogen bonds. These bonds are significantly weaker than the chemical bonds that involve sharing or transferring of electrons, and they have only 5 to 10 percent of the strength of a covalent bond.

Despite its relative weakness, hydrogen bonding is quite important in the natural world; it has major effects on the properties of water and ice and is important biologically with regard to proteins and nucleic acids as well as the DNA double-helix structure.

Van der Waals forces are electrical interactions between two or more molecules or atoms. They are the weakest type of intermolecular attraction, but their net effect can be quite strong. There are two major types of van der Waals forces. The **London dispersion force** is a temporary force that occurs when electrons in two adjacent atoms form spontaneous, temporary dipoles due to the positions the atoms are occupying. This is the weakest intermolecular force, and it does not exert a force over long distances.

The second type of van der Waals force is **dipole-dipole interactions**, which are the result of two dipolar molecules interacting with each other. This interaction occurs when the partial positive dipole in one molecule is attracted to the partial negative dipole in the other molecule.

PRACTICE QUESTION

13. The weak attraction between temporary dipoles creates

   A) the London dispersion force.

   B) a hydrogen bond.

   C) dipole-dipole interactions.

   D) a covalent bond.

Physical and Chemical Properties

Substances, whether they are composed of individual atoms or molecules, all have unique properties that are grouped into two categories: physical and chemical. A change in a **physical property** (called a physical change) results only in a change of the physical structure, not in the chemical composition of a reactant. For example, a change of state is a physical reaction. A physical property may be identified just by observing, touching, or measuring the substance in some way.

A change in a **chemical property** is one in which the molecular structure or composition of the compound has been changed. Chemical properties cannot be identified simply by observing a material. Rather, the material must be engaged in a chemical reaction in order to identify its chemical properties.

Physical and chemical properties are often influenced by intramolecular and intermolecular forces. For example, substances with strong hydrogen bonds will have higher boiling points.

TABLE 9.2. Physical and Chemical Properties	
PHYSICAL PROPERTIES	**CHEMICAL PROPERTIES**
temperature	heat of combustion
color	flammability
mass	toxicity
density	chemical stability
viscosity	enthalpy of formation

PRACTICE QUESTION

14. Which of the following describes a physical change?

A) Water becomes ice.

B) Batter is baked into a cake.

C) A firecracker explodes.

D) An acid is neutralized with a base.

States of Matter

A **state** (also called a phase) is a description of the physical characteristics of a material. There are four states: solid, liquid, gas, and plasma.

- A **solid** is a dense phase characterized by close bonds between all molecules in the solid; solids have a definite shape and volume.

- A **liquid** is a fluid phase characterized by loose bonds between molecules in the liquid; liquids have an indefinite shape but a definite volume.

- A **gas** is a very disperse phase characterized by the lack of, or very weak, bonds between molecules; gases have both an indefinite shape and volume.

- The **plasma** phase occurs when a substance has been heated and pressurized past its critical point, resulting in a new phase that has liquid and gas properties.

A substance will change phase depending on the temperature and pressure. As temperature increases, the phase will progress from solid to liquid to gas. As pressure increases, the opposite is true, and the phase will progress from gas to liquid to solid.

These phase changes have specific names, as shown below. Note that reciprocal changes will involve the same amount of energy; however, moving from a less to a more energetic state uses energy, while moving from a more to a less energetic state will release energy.

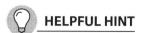
TABLE 9.3. Phase Changes

NAME	FROM	TO	OCCURS AT	ENERGY CHANGE
Evaporation	liquid	gas	boiling point	uses energy
Condensation	gas	liquid	boiling point	releases energy
Melting	solid	liquid	freezing point	uses energy
Freezing	liquid	solid	freezing point	releases energy
Sublimation	solid	gas	---	uses energy
Deposition	gas	solid	---	releases energy

Phase diagrams are used to show the relationships between phases, temperature, and pressure for a particular substance. In the phase diagram, there are two points that are interesting to note. At the **triple point**, all three phases exist together, and at the **critical point**, the substance enters the plasma phase.

The boiling point and freezing point of a molecule are related to its structure. There are three important factors that contribute to boiling and freezing points:

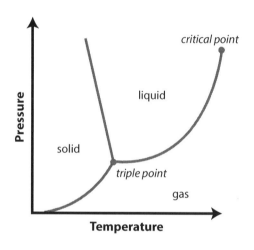

Figure 9.8. Phase Diagram

1. **Strength of intermolecular forces:** the greater the intermolecular force, the greater the substance's boiling point.

2. **Molecule size:** as the molecule becomes larger, the boiling point of the molecule typically increases.

3. **Molecule branching:** as more branch points are present in the molecule, the molecule's boiling point will decrease.

Methane has a molecular weight of 16 grams per mole, and water has a molecular weight of 18 grams per mole. Neither molecule is branched. As a result, factors 2 and 3 (as listed above) are not relevant. However, water has a boiling point of 100°C, while methane has a boiling point of −164°C.

This large difference is a result of intermolecular forces. Water is a highly polar molecule that has strong intermolecular forces. On the other hand, methane is an uncharged, nonpolar molecule with next to no intermolecular forces. Thus, the energy required to break the bonds between water molecules, and cause the phase change from liquid to vapor, is much greater than that for the methane molecule.

PRACTICE QUESTIONS

15. Which of the following is likely to have the highest number of molecules?

    A) 1 liter of gaseous CO_2

    B) 1 liter of liquid CO_2

    C) 1 liter of solid CO_2

    D) 1 liter of a mix of solid and gaseous CO_2

16. Which of the following terms describes the phase change from liquid to solid?

    A) evaporation

    B) deposition

    C) melting

    D) freezing

Properties of Water

Water has many unique properties that make it essential to life on Earth. Those properties are the result of its unique chemical composition and shape. Water has the formula H_2O and is held together by a polar covalent bond. The oxygen has a slightly negative charge, and the two hydrogen atoms have a slightly positive charge. Water's unique properties include:

- **cohesion**: Because of their polarity, water molecules are attracted to each other.

- **adhesion**: Water's polarity also causes it to cling to other substances.

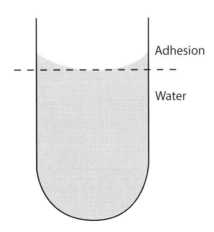

Figure 9.9. Adhesion

- **surface tension**: The molecules on the surface of water are highly attracted to each other, making it harder to puncture the surface.

- **capillary action**: The ability of water to move upward against gravity through narrow spaces (due to water's adhesion to surfaces).

- Water is a strong solvent that can dissolve many ionic compounds.

- Water has a low molecular weight but a high boiling and freezing point, making it the only compound on Earth found naturally in all three phases (gas, liquid, solid).

- Solid water (ice) forms a crystal lattice structure with widely spaced molecules, making ice less dense than liquid water. This property causes ice to float.

PRACTICE QUESTION

17. Which property of water allows plants to pull water up from their roots to their leaves?

A) surface tension

B) capillary action

C) low molecular weight

D) crystal lattice structure of ice

Acids and Bases

The Definition of Acids and Bases

In general, an **acid** can be defined as a substance that produces hydrogen ions (H^+) in solution, while a **base** produces hydroxide ions (OH^-). Acidic solutions, which include common liquids like orange juice and vinegar, share a set of distinct characteristics: they have a sour taste and react strongly with metals. Bases, such as bleach and detergents, will taste bitter and have a slippery texture.

There are a number of different technical definitions for acids and bases, including the Arrhenius, Brønsted-Lowry, and Lewis acid definitions.

- The **Arrhenius** definition: An acid is a substance that produces H^+ hydrogen ions in aqueous solution. A base is a substance that produces hydroxide ions OH^- in aqueous solution.

- The **Brønsted-Lowry** definition: An acid is anything that donates a proton H^+, and a base is anything that accepts a proton H^+.

- The **Lewis** definition: An acid is anything able to accept a pair of electrons, and a base is anything that can donate a pair of electrons.

18. Which of the following is a base?

    A) $Ba(OH)_2$

    B) HCl

    C) $HClO_4$

    D) HI

Measuring the Strength of Acids and Bases

The **pH** of a solution is a measure of the acidity or basicity of the solution. It is found by taking the negative log of the concentration of hydrogen ions, making pH an exponential scale:

$$pH = -\log[H^+]$$

The pH scale runs from 0 to 14 with a low pH being more acidic and a high pH being more basic. A pH of 7 is that of water with no dissolved ions and is considered neutral.

pH scale

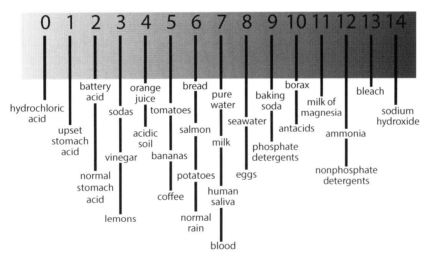

Figure 9.10. pH Scale

 HELPFUL HINT

A buffer is a chemical system that resists changes in pH when small quantities of acids or bases are added. The buffer contains a weak acid to react with any added base and a weak base to react with any added acid.

Strong acids and bases will dissolve completely in solution, while weak acids and bases will only partially dissolve. Thus, strong acids and bases will have high or low pH values, respectively, and weak acids and bases will have pH values closer to 7.

TABLE 9.4. Strong Acids and Bases

Strong acids	HCl	Hydrochloric acid
	HNO_3	Nitric acid
	H_2SO_4	Sulfuric acid
	$HClO_4$	Perchloric acid
	HBr	Hydrobromic acid
	HI	Hydroiodic acid
Strong bases	LiOH	Lithium hydroxide
	NaOH	Sodium hydroxide
	KOH	Potassium hydroxide
	$Ca(OH)_2$	Calcium hydroxide
	$Ba(OH)_2$	Barium hydroxide
	$Sr(OH)_2$	Strontium hydroxide

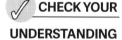

CHECK YOUR UNDERSTANDING

What acidic and basic solutions do you handle on a daily basis?

PRACTICE QUESTIONS

19. Which of the following best describes a substance with a pH of 12?

A) very acidic

B) slightly acidic

C) neutral

D) very basic

20. Which of the following acids is a strong acid?

A) HClO

B) HBr

C) HF

D) HN_3

Solutions

CHECK YOUR UNDERSTANDING

Are the following mixtures homogenous or heterogeneous?

lemonade, concrete, air, trail mix, salt water

In chemistry, the term **mixture** describes a set of two or more substances that have been mixed together but are not chemically joined together. In a **homogenous** mixture, the substances are evenly distributed; in a **heterogeneous** mixture, the substances are not evenly distributed.

A **solution** is a specific type of homogenous mixture in which all substances share the same basic properties and generally act as a single substance. In a solution, a **solute** is dissolved in a **solvent**. For example, in salt water, salt is the solute and water is the solvent. The opposite process, in which a compound comes out of the solution, is called **precipitation**.

The **concentration** of a solution—the amount of solute versus the amount of solvent—can be measured in a number of ways. Usually it is given as a ratio of solute to solvent in the relevant units. Some of these include:

- moles per volume (e.g., moles per liter)—also called **molarity**

- moles per mass (e.g., moles per kilogram)—also called **molality**

- mass per volume (e.g., grams per liter)

- volume per volume (e.g., milliliters per liter)

- mass per mass (e.g., milligrams per gram)

Solubility is a measure of how much solute will dissolve into a solvent. When a solution contains the maximum amount of solute possible, it is called a **saturated solution**. A solution with less solute is **unsaturated**, and a solution with more solute than can normally be dissolved in that solvent is **supersaturated**.

There are many factors that can affect the solubility of a compound, including temperature and pressure. Generally, solubility increases with temperature (although there are some compounds whose solubility will decrease with an increase in temperature). The relationship between solubility and temperature is shown in a solubility curve.

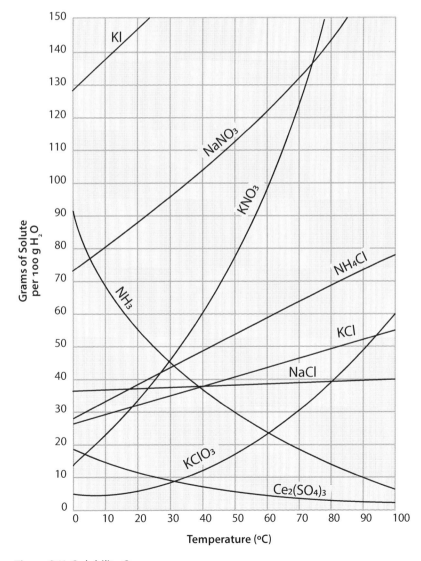

Figure 9.11. Solubility Curve

Another factor affecting solubility is the **common ion effect**, which occurs in solutions with two compounds that share a common ion. When the two compounds are mixed into a solvent, the presence of the common ion reduces the solubility of each compound. For example, $NaCl$ and $MgCl_2$ share the common ion of chlorine. When they are mixed in a solution, the maximum saturation of the chlorine ion in water will be reached before the saturation of either sodium or magnesium is reached. This causes a reduction in the overall solubility.

PRACTICE QUESTIONS

21. In a carbonated soda, carbon dioxide is dissolved in water. Which of the following terms describes the water in this mixture?

    A) common ion

    B) solvent

    C) solute

    D) precipitant

22. Which of the following terms describes a solution in which more solvent can be dissolved?

    A) unsaturated

    B) saturated

    C) supersaturated

    D) homogenous

Chemical Reactions

The Nature of Chemical Reactions

In a **chemical reaction**, one set of chemical substances, called the **reactants**, is transformed into another set of chemical substances, called the **products**. This transformation is described in a chemical equation with the reactants on the left and products on the right. In the equation below, methane (CH_4) reacts with oxygen (O_2) to produce carbon dioxide (CO_2) and water (H_2O).

$$CH_4 + 2O_2 \rightarrow CO_2 + 2H_2O$$

When a reaction runs to **completion**, all the reactants have been used up in the reaction. If one reactant limits the use of the other reactants (i.e., if one reactant is used up before the others), it is called the **limiting reactant**. The **yield** is the amount of product produced by the reaction.

A chemical reaction that uses energy is **endothermic**, while a reaction that releases energy is **exothermic**. Generally, creating bonds requires energy, and breaking bonds releases energy. Whether a reaction is endothermic or exothermic depends on the specific energy requirements of the bonds being broken and made in the reaction.

Processes can also be described as being endothermic or exothermic. For example, boiling water to form vapor is an endothermic process because it requires energy. Freezing liquid water to form ice is an exothermic process because it releases energy.

PRACTICE QUESTION

23. An exothermic reaction will always

   A) run to completion.

   B) have a limiting reagent.

   C) release energy.

   D) use energy.

Balancing Equations

The integer values placed before the chemical symbols are the **coefficients** that describe how many molecules of that substance are involved in the reaction. These values are important because in a chemical reaction, there is a **conservation of mass**: the number and type of atoms in the reactants must match the number and type of atoms in the products.

In order to **balance an equation**, you'll need to add the coefficients necessary to match the atoms of each element on both sides. In the reaction below, the numbers of bromine (Br) and nitrate ions (NO_3^-) do not match up:

$$CaBr_2 + NaNO_3 \rightarrow Ca(NO_3)_2 + NaBr$$

To balance the equation, start by adding a coefficient of 2 to the products to balance the bromine:

$$CaBr_2 + NaNO_3 \rightarrow Ca(NO_3)_2 + 2NaBr$$

There are now 2 sodium ions on the right, so another 2 need to be added on the left to balance it:

$$CaBr_2 + 2NaNO_3 \rightarrow Ca(NO_3)_2 + 2NaBr$$

Notice that adding this 2 also balances the nitrate ions, so the equation is now complete.

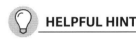 **HELPFUL HINT**

Always balance H and O last when balancing chemical equations.

PRACTICE QUESTION

24. Which of the following equations is a balanced equation?

   A) $2KClO_3 \rightarrow KCl + 3O_2$

   B) $KClO_3 \rightarrow KCl + 3O_2$

   C) $2KClO_3 \rightarrow 2KCl + 3O_2$

   D) $6KClO_3 \rightarrow 6KCl + 3O_2$

Moles

A **mole (mol)** is the SI unit for the amount of a substance. One mole of an element contains 6.02×10^{23} atoms of that element. One mole of a compound contains 6.02×10^{23} of each atom in that compound.

$$1 \text{ mole C} = 6.02 \times 10^{23} \text{ C atoms}$$

$$1 \text{ mole CH}_4 = 6.02 \times 10^{23} \text{ C atoms and } 4(6.02 \times 10^{23}) \text{ H atoms}$$

The weight of a mole of an element or compound is called its **molar mass**. A mole of an element weighs the same in grams as the atomic weight (in amu). For example, a mole of carbon weighs 12.01 g. The molar mass of a compound is found by adding the molar mass of each atom in the compound.

$$\text{molar mass H}_2\text{O} = 2(1 \text{ g}) + 16 \text{ g} = 18 \text{ g}$$

The molar mass of an element or compound can be used as a conversion factor to convert between moles and grams.

$$\frac{3 \text{ g C}}{} \quad \frac{1 \text{ mol}}{12.01 \text{ g}} = 0.25 \text{ mol C}$$

$$\frac{5 \text{ mol O}_2}{} \quad \frac{32 \text{ g}}{1 \text{ mol}} = 160 \text{ g O}_2$$

The coefficients in a chemical reaction correspond to the number of moles of each substance involved in the reaction. The combustion of methane (shown below) requires 1 mole of methane and 2 moles of oxygen gas; it produces 1 mole of carbon dioxide and 2 moles of water.

$$CH_4 \ (g) + 2O_2 \ (g) \rightarrow CO_2 \ (g) + 2H_2O \ (l)$$

The weight of substances involved in a reaction can be found using their molar mass and the reaction equation. The example below shows the weight of the reactants and products involved when 1 mole of methane combusts with unlimited oxygen.

$$CH_4 \ (g) + 2O_2 \ (g) \rightarrow CO_2 \ (g) + 2H_2O \ (l)$$

Reactants

$$\frac{1 \text{ mol CH}_4}{} \quad \frac{16 \text{ g}}{1 \text{ mol}} = 16 \text{ g CH}_4$$

$$\frac{2 \text{ mol O}_2}{} \quad \frac{32 \text{ g}}{1 \text{ mol}} = 64 \text{ g O}_2$$

$$\begin{array}{c|c|c}
\text{1 mol CO}_2 & \dfrac{44\ \text{g}}{1\ \text{mol}} & = 44\ \text{g CO}_2
\end{array}$$

$$\begin{array}{c|c|c}
\text{2 mol H}_2\text{O} & \dfrac{18\ \text{g}}{1\ \text{mol}} & = 36\ \text{g H}_2\text{O}
\end{array}$$

Products

PRACTICE QUESTION

25. How many moles of NaCl are in 5 g of NaCl?

A) 0.09 mol

B) 11.69 mol

C) 3.01×10^{24} mol

D) 8.31×10^{-24} mol

Types of Reactions

There are five main types of chemical reactions. In a **synthesis reaction**, two reactants combine to form a single product. A **decomposition reaction** is the opposite of a synthesis reaction and involves a single reactant breaking down into several products.

In a displacement reaction, one ion takes the place of another in a compound. **Single-displacement** reactions include a free ion taking the place of the ion in a compound. In a **double-displacement** reaction, ions in two different compounds switch places.

Finally, in a **combustion reaction**, a fuel (usually an alkane or carbohydrate) will react with oxygen to form carbon dioxide and water. Combustion reactions also produce heat.

The five types of chemical reactions are summarized in Table 9.5.

TABLE 9.5. Types of Reactions

TYPE OF REACTION	GENERAL FORMULA	EXAMPLE REACTION
Synthesis	$A + B \rightarrow C$	$2H_2 + O_2 \rightarrow 2H_2O$
Decomposition	$A \rightarrow B + C$	$2H_2O_2 \rightarrow 2H_2O + O_2$
Single displacement	$AB + C \rightarrow A + BC$	$CH_4 + Cl_2 \rightarrow CH_3Cl + HCl$
Double displacement	$AB + CD \rightarrow AC + BD$	$CuCl_2 + 2AgNO_3 \rightarrow Cu(NO_3)_2 + 2AgCl$
Combustion	$C_xH_yO_z + O_2 \rightarrow CO_2 + H_2O$	$2C_8H_{18} + 25O_2 \rightarrow 16CO_2 + 18H_2O$

Neutralization is a specific type of double-displacement reaction in which an acid and base react to form a salt and water. As a result of this reaction, if an equal amount of strong acid is mixed with an equal amount of strong base, the pH will remain at 7. For example, mixing hydrochloric acid and sodium hydroxide yields sodium chloride (a salt) and water, as shown below:

$$HCl + Na(OH) \rightarrow H_2O + NaCl$$

PRACTICE QUESTION

26. Which of the following types of reactions is shown below?

$Pb(NO_3)_2 + K_2CrO_4 \rightarrow PbCrO_4 + 2\ KNO_3$

A) combustion

B) decomposition

C) double displacement

D) single replacement

Oxidation and Reduction Reactions

An oxidation and reduction reaction (often called a redox reaction) is one in which there is an exchange of electrons. The species that loses electrons is **oxidized**, and the species that gains electrons is **reduced**. The species that loses electrons is also called the **reducing agent**, and the species that gains electrons is the **oxidizing agent**.

The movement of electrons in a redox reaction is analyzed by assigning each atom in the reaction an **oxidation number** (or state) that corresponds roughly to that atom's charge. (The actual meaning of the oxidation number is much more complicated.) Once all the atoms in a reaction have been assigned an oxidation number, it is possible to see which elements have gained electrons and which elements have lost electrons. The basic rules for assigning oxidation numbers are given in the table below.

TABLE 9.6. Assigning Oxidation Numbers

SPECIES	EXAMPLE	OXIDATION NUMBER
Elements in their free state and naturally occurring diatomic elements	$Zn(s)$, O_2	0
Monoatomic ions	Cl^-	-1
Oxygen in compounds	H_2O	-2
Hydrogen in compounds	HCl	$+1$
Alkali metals in a compound	Na	$+1$
Alkaline earth metals in a compound	Mg	$+2$
RULES		
The oxidation numbers on the atoms in a neutral compound sum to zero.	NaOH	Na: $+1$; O: -2; H: $+1$ $1 + -2 + 1 = 0$
The oxidation numbers of the atoms in an ion sum to the charge on that ion.	SO_3^{-2}	S: $+4$; O: -2 $4 + (-2)(3) = -2$

PRACTICE QUESTION

27. Which of the following substances is reduced in the reaction shown below?

$$Fe_2O_3 + 3CO \rightarrow 2Fe + 3CO_2$$

A) Fe

B) O

C) CO

D) CO_2

Collision Theory and Reaction Rates

Collision theory refers to the idea that a chemical reaction cannot occur until two molecules that may react collide with one another. In a solid, although molecules are all touching one another, there is not much movement. As a result, chemical reactions in solid phase have a low reaction rate or none at all. A solid usually reacts only when its surface comes into contact with a liquid or gas.

In liquids or gases, molecules are able to move freely, which allows greater interaction and an increased chance that two capable molecules will react. For this reason, the majority of chemical reactions occur in the liquid phase or the gas phase. However, even if two molecules collide that could react, most of the time they do not. In order for a reaction to take place, the reaction must have a minimum amount of energy, a quantity known as the reaction's **activation energy**.

Different reactions will occur at different rates. This **reaction rate** is determined by a number of factors, including the concentration of reactants, particle surface area, and temperature. Generally, increasing any of these variables will increase the reaction rate by providing more opportunities for particles to collide.

- Increasing the concentration of reactants introduces more particles to the system, meaning they are more likely to collide.

- Increasing particle surface area makes it more likely particles will come in contact with each other.

- Increasing the temperature increases the velocity of the particles, making them more likely to collide.

PRACTICE QUESTION

28. Which of the following describes the effect of increasing the concentration of the reactants in a reaction?

A) The reaction rate will increase.

B) The reaction rate will decrease.

C) The change in the reaction rate will depend on the temperature of the reaction.

D) The change in the reaction rate will depend on the pressure of the reaction.

Catalysts

Substances called **catalysts** increase reaction rates by providing an alternative pathway with a lower activation energy. Catalysts themselves are unchanged during the chemical reaction. A chemical catalyst is commonly a metal or other elemental compound with many electrons in its valence shell; catalysts assist in the stabilization of reaction intermediates. Common chemical catalysts include platinum, palladium, nickel, and cobalt.

A biological catalyst is known as an **enzyme**. Common enzymes include cellulase, amylase, or DNA polymerase. Biological catalysts typically function by bringing two reactants close together and are usually designed to catalyze a specific reaction. This specificity is referred to as the **lock and key model**: most keys can only open specific locks. Similarly, the shape of any one enzyme only matches the shape of the molecule it reacts with, called a **substrate**. The **active site** is the place on the enzyme that directly contacts the substrate, or the place where the two "puzzle pieces" fit together, facilitating the actual reaction.

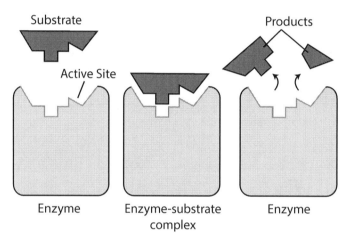

Figure 9.12. Enzyme Function

There are two types of catalysts subdivided by their phase: homogenous and heterogeneous. A **homogenous catalyst** is in the same phase as the reactants. Most enzymes are homogenous and are soluble in the same phase as the reactants.

A **heterogeneous catalyst** is not in the same phase as the reactants. An example of a heterogeneous catalyst is the platinum found in the catalytic converter in the exhaust stream of cars. The catalyst is in the solid phase, and the reactants are in the gas phase.

PRACTICE QUESTION

29. Which of the following best describes the role of a catalyst in a reaction?

A) A catalyst increases the activation energy required for a reaction to take place.

B) A catalyst increases the rate at which reactants become products.

C) A catalyst shifts the reaction toward the reactants.

D) A catalyst increases the amount of product produced.

Chemical Equilibria

A **chemical equilibrium** occurs when the concentrations of reactants and products remain constant in a reaction system. This does not mean that the chemical reaction has stopped, just that the forward and backward reactions are occurring at equal rates. Chemical equilibria are represented in equations with a double arrow. An example of a system in chemical equilibrium is a weak acid, which only partially ionizes (breaks apart) in water.

$$CH_3COOH\ (aq) + H_2O\ (l) \leftrightarrow CH_3COO^-\ (aq) + H_3O^+\ (aq)$$

While more than 90 percent of the acid remains in its molecular form (CH_3COOH) at equilibrium, both the forward and backward reactions are occurring at the same rates.

Changing the condition of a reaction can change the balance of reactants and products. **Le Châtelier's principle** states that if a chemical reaction system is at equilibrium, and the conditions are changed so it is no longer at equilibrium, the system will react to counteract the change and reach a new equilibrium. Applying changes to a system in equilibrium is known as *shifting the equilibrium*. The equilibrium can shift to either the right (forward direction, products) or left (reverse direction, reactants). Some of these changes are summarized in Table 9.7.

TABLE 9.7. Le Châtelier's Principle

CHANGE	SHIFT
Increase in reaction concentration	to products
Increase in product concentration	to reactants
Increase pressure *or* Decrease volume	toward fewer moles of gas
Decrease pressure *or* Increase volume	toward more moles of gas
Increase temperature	toward endothermic direction
Decrease temperature	toward exothermic direction
Addition of catalyst	no shift

HELPFUL HINT

Chemical equilibria are not affected by catalysts. Catalysts can speed up the rate at which equilibrium is achieved, but they cannot change the equilibrium concentrations.

CHECK YOUR UNDERSTANDING

Transferring gas into and out of the blood is an equilibrium process. For oxygen, it is represented by $Hb_4 + 4O_2 \leftrightarrow Hb_4O_8$, where Hb is hemoglobin. How would this reaction maintain equilibrium when it occurs (1) in the lungs with high oxygen concentration and (2) near tissues with low oxygen concentration?

PRACTICE QUESTION

30. The following reaction is in equilibrium:

$BaSO_4\ (s) \leftrightarrow Ba^{2+}\ (aq) + SO_4^{2-}\ (aq)$

What will happen to the concentration of Ba^{2+} if more $BaSO_4$ is added to the reaction?

A) It will increase.

B) It will decrease.

C) There will be no change.

D) There is insufficient information to determine the effect.

---

1. **C)** The nucleus of an atom includes protons and neutrons. Electrons orbit around the nucleus.

2. **D)** The total charge of an atom is calculated by the difference between the number of protons and electrons: $5 - 7 = -2$.

3. **A)** Phosphorus has fifteen electrons. Filling the orbitals from lowest to highest energy (as shown in Figure 9.2.) gives the electron configuration $1s^2 2s^2 2p^6 3s^2 3p^3$.

4. **A)** The valence shell of the noble gases, group 18, is full, so they do not need any electrons to complete them.

5. **D)** *atomic mass − atomic number = number of neutrons*

6. **C)** The elements F, Cl, and Br are halogens in group 17 and thus have seven electrons in their valence shells.

7. **A)** Sodium (Na) is in group 1, the alkali metals.

8. **D)** Both Se and O are found in group 16, so they have six electrons in their valence shell. They will add two electrons to fill the shell, resulting in a charge of −2.

9. **D)** Electronegativity increases from left to right and bottom to top on the periodic table, with fluorine (F) being the most electronegative element.

10. **A)** All of these elements are in the same period. Atomic radius decreases from left to right across the periodic table; since oxygen (O) is the element farthest to the right in the period, it will have the smallest atomic radius.

11. **C)** Fluorine is more electronegative than carbon (C), oxygen (O), or nitrogen (N). In the bond with hydrogen, it will pull the shared electrons more strongly, creating the bond with the highest polarity.

12. **B)** Calcium is an alkaline earth metal and easily forms a +2 cation, which in turn forms an ionic bond with an anion. Argon is a noble gas and does not form bonds, and copper is a metal that forms metallic bonds. Nitrogen most often forms covalent bonds.

13. **A)** The London dispersion force is a temporary force that occurs when electrons in two adjacent atoms form spontaneous, temporary dipoles.

14. **A)** When water changes states, its chemical composition does not change. Once water becomes ice, the ice can easily turn back into water.

15. **C)** Molecules are more closely packed together in a solid than in a liquid or gas. So, 1 L of solid CO_2 would have more molecules than 1 L of gaseous or liquid CO_2.

16. **D)** Freezing is the change from liquid to solid, as when liquid water freezes to form solid ice.

17. **B)** Plants use capillary action to move water through narrow vessels from their roots to their leaves.

18. **A)** $Ba(OH)_2$ is a base; bases usually include a hydroxide ion (OH).

19. **D)** Substances with a pH higher than 7 are basic. The pH scale goes up to 14, meaning a pH of 12 is very basic.

20. **B)** Hydrobromic acid (HBr) is one of the strong acids.

21. **B)** The water is the solvent in which the solute (carbon dioxide) is dissolved.

22. **A)** An unsaturated solution has less solute than can be dissolved in the given amount of solvent.

23. **C)** Exothermic reactions release energy.

24. **C)** In this equation, there are equal numbers of each type of atom on both sides (2 K atoms, 2 Cl atoms, and 6 O atoms).

25. **A)** Find the molar mass of NaCl and use dimensional analysis.
    Na: 22.99 g
    Cl: 35.45 g
    NaCl: 22.99 + 35.45 = 58.44 g

5 g	1 mol	= 0.09 mol
	58.44 g	

26. **C)** In the reaction, the Pb and K exchange their anions in a double-displacement reaction.

27. **A)** Fe has an oxidation number of +3 in the compound Fe_2O_3 and an oxidation number of 0 on its own as Fe. Because Fe lost three electrons (to go from +3 to 0), it was reduced.

28. **A)** A higher concentration of reactants increases the rate of reaction by increasing the number of collisions between reactant molecules.

29. **B)** A catalyst increases the rate of a reaction by providing an alternative path for the reaction that has a lower activation energy.

30. **A)** Adding more reactants will push the reaction forward toward the products to reach a new equilibrium, which will increase the amount of each product.

10 | Scientific Reasoning

Systems

A **system** is a set of interacting parts that work together to form an integrated whole. Many scientific disciplines study systems: doctors, for example, study organ systems like the respiratory system, which is made up of interacting parts that allow animals to breathe. Similarly, ecologists might look at all the plants and animals that interact in a specific area, and chemists might look at a set of chemicals interacting in a beaker. While obviously different, all these systems share some common traits.

TABLE 10.1. Characteristics of Systems

CHARACTERISTIC	EXAMPLE (RESPIRATORY SYSTEM)
All systems have a structure.	The respiratory system is highly organized.
All systems perform an action.	The respiratory system allows animals to breathe.
All systems have interacting parts.	The respiratory system is made up of many interacting parts, including the lungs, blood vessels, and bronchial tubes.
All systems have boundaries.	We can separate structures that are part of the respiratory system from those that are not.
Systems may receive input and produce output.	The respiratory system brings oxygen into the body and gets rid of carbon dioxide.
The processes in a system may be controlled by feedback.	The action of breathing is controlled in part by how much oxygen and carbon dioxide are in the body.

Sometimes larger systems are made of smaller, independent systems called **subsystems**. For example, a cell is made of many organelles. These organelles each perform their own tasks, which together support the system of the cell.

Scientific Investigations

Although science can never definitively "prove" something, it does provide a means to answering many questions about our natural world. The scientific process starts with **observations**, the recording of aspects of the natural world. Observations can be quantitative or qualitative.

- **Quantitative** observations can be measured (e.g., number, length, mass, volume).

- **Qualitative** observations cannot be measured (e.g., color, shape, texture).

Observations lead scientists to ask questions, and then an **investigation** can be designed to answer that question. Scientists use different types of investigations, each providing different types of results, based upon what they are trying to find. There are three main types of scientific investigations: experimental, descriptive, and comparative.

Experimental investigations are designed to test a **hypothesis**, which is a proposed explanation for a phenomenon based on observations or previous research. In an experimental investigation, an **independent variable** is manipulated, and the **dependent variable** is measured. Other factors that might affect the dependent variable, called **control variables**, are held constant throughout the experiment.

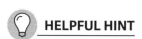 **HELPFUL HINT**

A hypothesis is more than an educated guess. Instead, a hypothesis is a testable proposition that scientists can use as the basis for an investigation. If it is not capable of being tested scientifically, it is not a hypothesis.

TABLE 10.2. Parts of an Experimental Investigation

PART	WHAT IS IT?	EXAMPLE
Hypothesis	a proposed explanation for a phenomenon	People who increase the amount of cardiovascular exercise they do will lose weight.
Independent variable	the variable being manipulated	amount of cardiovascular exercise
Dependent variable	the variable being measured	weight
Control variables	variables that may affect the dependent variable that are held constant	diet of subjects type of cardiovascular exercise initial weight of subjects

Descriptive investigations start with observations. A model is then constructed to provide a visual of what was seen: a description. Descriptive investigations do not generally require hypotheses, as they usually just attempt to find more information about a relatively unknown topic.

Lastly, **comparative investigations** involve manipulating different groups in order to compare them with each other. There is no control during comparative investigations.

Laws and Theories

Once a hypothesis has been thoroughly tested and is generally accepted to be true in the scientific community, it can be incorporated into the existing body of scientific knowledge. This body of knowledge includes facts, laws, and theories. A **fact** is simply an observation that is accepted as "true" by the scientific community. A **law** is a statement that describes how aspects of the natural world behave under specific circumstances. Finally, a **theory** is an accepted explanation for a natural phenomenon.

TABLE 10.3. Types of Scientific Knowledge

TERM	WHAT IS IT?	EXAMPLE
Fact	an observation that is accepted as true	Genes code for proteins.
Law	a statement that describes how nature behaves	Mendel's law of independent assortment
Theory	an accepted explanation for a natural phenomenon	theory of evolution

Sources of Error

When designing an experiment, scientists must identify possible sources of error. These can be **confounding variables**, which are factors that act like the independent variable and thus can make it appear that the independent variable has a greater effect than it actually does. The design may also include unknown variables that are not controlled by the scientists. Finally, scientists must be aware of **human error**, particularly in collecting data and making observations, and of possible equipment errors.

The Scientific Method

In order to ensure that experimental and comparative investigations are thorough and accurate, scientists use the scientific method, which has five main steps:

1. Observe and ask questions: look at the natural world to observe and ask questions about patterns and anomalies you see.

2. Gather information: look at what other scientists have done to see where your questions fit in with current research.

3. Construct a hypothesis: make a proposal that explains why or how something happens.

4. Experiment and test your hypothesis: set up an experimental investigation that allows you to test your hypothesis.

5. Analyze results and draw conclusions: examine your results and see whether they disprove your hypothesis. Note that you can't actually *prove* a hypothesis; you can only provide evidence to support it.

PRACTICE QUESTIONS

1. Which of the following BEST defines a hypothesis?

   A) an educated guess

   B) a study of the natural world

   C) an explanation of a natural phenomenon

   D) a testable proposed scientific explanation

2. A student wants to find out if the time of day she takes an exam affects the score she receives. She gathers together all the tests she took in her algebra, biology, and world history classes during the last year and records the time she took the exam and the score she received. Which of the following is the dependent variable in her investigation?

   A) the time she took an exam

   B) the subject of the exam

   C) the score she received on an exam

   D) the number of exams she took

3. Which of the following correctly describes a scientific theory?

   A) a proposed explanation for an observation in nature

   B) an explanation for natural phenomena that has not been refuted despite multiple tests

   C) specific observations that have been documented by multiple sources

   D) a conjecture that is based on limited information

4. Why is the germ theory of disease considered to be a theory?

   A) There is insufficient evidence to support it.

   B) Valid alternative explanations exist.

   C) It is strongly supported by existing evidence.

   D) It has only limited clinical application.

5. A scientist is observing the flower of a new plant species. Which of the following information collected by the scientist is qualitative data?

   A) color of the flower petals

   B) height of the flower

   C) time of day the flower opened

   D) number of petals on the flower

Answer Key

1. **D)** A hypothesis must be testable and propose an explanation of observed natural phenomena.

2. **C)** She wants to see if time of day (the independent variable) affects her exam scores (the dependent variable).

3. **B)** Scientific theories are explanatory in nature and are supported by a large accumulation of data in the scientific community.

4. **C)** A scientific theory is typically strongly supported by evidence, despite public misunderstanding to the contrary.

5. **A)** Qualitative data describes qualities that are not numerical and cannot be measured, such as color.

The English and Language Usage section will test your understanding of the basic rules of grammar. The good news is that you have been using these rules since you first began to speak. Even if you do not know a lot of the technical terms, many of these rules will be familiar to you. Some of the topics you might see include:

- matching pronouns with their antecedents
- matching verbs with their subjects
- ensuring that verbs are in the correct tense
- spelling irregular, hyphenated, and commonly misspelled words
- using correct capitalization
- distinguishing between types of sentences
- correcting sentence structure

11 Parts of Speech

Nouns and Pronouns

Nouns are people, places, or things. The subject of a sentence is typically a noun. For example, in the sentence "The hospital was very clean," the subject, *hospital*, is a noun; it is a place. **Pronouns** stand in for nouns and can be used to make sentences sound less repetitive. Take the sentence "Sam stayed home from school because Sam was not feeling well." The name *Sam* appears twice in the same sentence. Instead of repeating the name, you can use the pronoun *he* to stand in for *Sam* and say, "Sam stayed home from school because he was not feeling well."

Because pronouns take the place of nouns, they need to agree in number with the noun they replace.

> The <u>teachers</u> are going to have a pizza party for <u>their</u> students.

Traditionally, pronouns must also agree in gender with the noun they are replacing; however this rule has become less stringent in recent years as ideas about gender identification continue to shift. The intentional use of *they* when referring to a singular noun is becoming more commonplace and accepted. Alternatively, sentences can be rewritten to avoid the use of gender-specific pronouns.

> **Traditional**: If a student forgets his or her homework, he or she will not receive a grade.
> **Use of singular *they***: If a student forgets their homework, they will not receive a grade.
> **Rewritten with a plural antecedent**: Students who forget their homework will not receive a grade.

Pronouns should also be used carefully to avoid ambiguity in sentences. In the example below, it's unclear who *she* refers to. The sentence needs to be rewritten for clarity:

 HELPFUL HINT

Singular Pronouns
I, me, my, mine
you, your, yours
he, him, his
she, her, hers
it, its
Plural Pronouns
we, us, our, ours
they, them, their, theirs

> **Incorrect**: After the teacher spoke to the student, she realized her mistake.
>
> **Correct**: After Mr. White spoke to the student, she realized her mistake.
>
> (*She* and *her* refer to the student.)
>
> **Correct**: After speaking to the student, the teacher realized her own mistake.
>
> (*Her* refers to the teacher.)

⚡⚡⚡⚡⚡PRACTICE QUESTIONS

I have lived in Minnesota since August, but I still don't own a warm coat or gloves.

1. Which of the following lists includes all the nouns in the sentence?

   A) coat, gloves

   B) I, coat, gloves

   C) Minnesota, August, coat, gloves

   D) I, Minnesota, August, warm, coat, gloves

2. In which of the following sentences do the nouns and pronouns NOT agree?

   A) After we walked inside, we took off our hats and shoes and put them in the closet.

   B) The members of the band should leave her instruments in the rehearsal room.

   C) The janitor on duty should rinse out his or her mop before leaving for the day.

   D) When you see someone in trouble, you should always try to help them.

Verbs

A **verb** is the action of a sentence: it describes what the subject of the sentence is or is doing. Verbs must match the subject of the sentence in person and number, and must be in the proper tense—past, present, or future.

Person describes the relationship of the speaker to the subject of the sentence: first (*I*, *we*), second (*you*), and third (*he*, *she*, *it*, *they*). **Number** refers to whether the subject of the sentence is singular or plural. Verbs are conjugated to match the person and number of the subject.

TABLE 11.1. Conjugating Verbs for Person

PERSON	SINGULAR	PLURAL
First	I jump	we jump
Second	you jump	you jump
Third	he/she/it jumps	they jump

> Wrong: The cat chase the ball while the dogs runs in the yard.
>
> Correct: The cat chases the ball while the dogs run in the yard.

Cat is singular, so it takes a singular verb (*chases*, which confusingly ends with an *s*); *dogs* is plural, so it needs a plural verb (*run*).

> Wrong: The cars that had been recalled by the manufacturer was returned within a few months.
>
> Correct: The cars that had been recalled by the manufacturer were returned within a few months.

Sometimes, the subject and verb are separated by clauses or phrases. In the above example, the subject *cars* is separated from the verb by the relatively long phrase "that had been recalled by the manufacturer," making it more difficult to determine how to correctly conjugate the verb.

> Correct: The doctor and nurse work in the hospital.
>
> Correct: Neither the nurse nor her boss was scheduled to take a vacation.
>
> Correct: Either the patient or her parents need to sign the release forms.

When the subject contains two or more nouns connected by *and*, that subject becomes plural and requires a plural verb. Singular subjects joined by *either/or*, *neither/nor*, or *not only/but also* remain singular; when these words join plural and singular subjects, the verb should match the closest subject.

Finally, verbs must be conjugated for tense, which shows when the action happened. Some conjugations include helping verbs like *was*, *have*, *have been*, and *will have been*.

TABLE 11.2. Verb Tenses

TENSE	PAST	PRESENT	FUTURE
Simple	I <u>gave</u> her a gift yesterday.	I <u>give</u> her a gift every day.	I <u>will give</u> her a gift on her birthday.
Continuous	I <u>was giving</u> her a gift when you got here.	I <u>am giving</u> her a gift; come in!	I <u>will be giving</u> her a gift at dinner.
Perfect	I <u>had given</u> her a gift before you got there.	I <u>have given</u> her a gift already.	I <u>will have given</u> her a gift by midnight.
Perfect continuous	Her friends <u>had been giving</u> her gifts all night when I arrived.	I <u>have been giving</u> her gifts every year for nine years.	I <u>will have been giving</u> her gifts on holidays for ten years next year.

 HELPFUL HINT

Think of the subject and the verb as sharing a single *s*. If the subject ends with an *s*, the verb should not, and vice versa.

 HELPFUL HINT

If the subject is separated from the verb, cross out the phrases between them to make conjugation easier.

→
CONTINUE

Tense must also be consistent throughout the sentence and the passage. For example, the sentence "I was baking cookies and eat some dough" sounds strange. That is because the two verbs, *was baking* and *eat*, are in different tenses. *Was baking* occurred in the past; *eat*, on the other hand, occurs in the present. To make them consistent, change *eat* to *ate*.

> Wrong: Because it will rain during the party last night, we had to move the tables inside.
>
> Correct: Because it rained during the party last night, we had to move the tables inside.

All the verb tenses in a sentence need to agree both with each other and with the other information in the sentence. In the first sentence above, the tense does not match the other information in the sentence: *last night* indicates the past (*rained*), not the future (*will rain*).

PRACTICE QUESTIONS

3. Which of the following sentences contains an incorrectly conjugated verb?

    A) The brother and sister runs very fast.

    B) Neither Anne nor Suzy likes the soup.

    C) The mother and father love their new baby.

    D) Either Jack or Jill will pick up the pizza.

4. Which of the following sentences contains an incorrect verb tense?

    A) After the show ended, we drove to the restaurant for dinner.

    B) Anne went to the mall before she headed home.

    C) Johnny went to the movies after he cleans the kitchen.

    D) Before the alarm sounded, smoke filled the cafeteria.

Adjectives and Adverbs

Adjectives provide more information about a noun in a sentence. Take the sentence "The boy hit the ball." If you want your readers to know more about the noun *boy*, you could use an adjective to describe him: *the little boy, the young boy, the tall boy*.

Adverbs and adjectives are similar because they provide more information about a part of a sentence. However, adverbs do not describe nouns—that's an adjective's job. Instead, adverbs describe verbs, adjectives, and even other adverbs. For example, in the sentence "The doctor had recently hired a new employee," the adverb *recently* tells us more about how the action *hired* took place.

Adjectives, adverbs, and **modifying phrases** (groups of words that together modify another word) should be placed as close as possible to the word they modify. Separating words from their modifiers can create incorrect or confusing sentences.

> Wrong: Running through the hall, the bell rang and the student knew she was late.
>
> Correct: Running through the hall, the student heard the bell ring and knew she was late.

The phrase *running through the hall* should be placed next to *student*, the noun it modifies.

> Wrong: Of my two friends, Clara is the smartest.
>
> Correct: Of my two friends, Clara is smarter.

The suffixes *−er* and *−est* are often used to modify adjectives when a sentence is making a comparison. The suffix *−er* is used when comparing two things, and the suffix *−est* is used when comparing more than two.

> Anne is taller than Steve, but Steve is more coordinated.
>
> Of the five brothers, Billy is the funniest, and Alex is the most intelligent.

Adjectives longer than two syllables are compared using *more* (for two things) or *most* (for three or more things).

> Wrong: My most warmest sweater is made of wool.
>
> Correct: My warmest sweater is made of wool.

More and *most* should not be used in conjunction with *−er* and *−est* endings.

PRACTICE QUESTIONS

The new chef carefully stirred the boiling soup and then lowered the heat.

5. Which of the following lists includes all the adjectives in the sentence?
   A) new, boiling
   B) new, carefully, boiling
   C) new, carefully, boiling, heat
   D) new, carefully, boiling, lowered, heat

6. Which of the following sentences contains an adjective error?
   A) The new red car was faster than the old blue car.
   B) Reggie's apartment is in the tallest building on the block.
   C) The slice of cake was tastier than the brownie.
   D) Of the four speeches, Jerry's was the most long.

→

CONTINUE

Other Parts of Speech

Prepositions express the location of a noun or pronoun in relation to other words and phrases in a sentence. For example, in the sentence "The nurse parked her car in a parking garage," the preposition *in* describes the position of the car in relation to the garage. Together, the preposition and the noun that follows it are called a **prepositional phrase**. In this example, the prepositional phrase is "in a parking garage."

Conjunctions connect words, phrases, and clauses. The conjunctions represented by the acronym FANBOYS—For, And, Nor, But, Or, Yet, So—are called **coordinating conjunctions** and are used to join **independent clauses** (clauses that can stand alone as a complete sentence). For example, in the following sentence, the conjunction *and* joins together two independent clauses:

> The nurse prepared the patient for surgery, and the doctor performed the surgery.

Other conjunctions, like *although*, *because*, and *if*, join together an independent and **dependent clause** (which cannot stand on its own). Take the following sentence:

> She had to ride the subway because her car was broken.

The clause "because her car was broken" cannot stand on its own.

Interjections, like *wow* and *hey*, express emotion and are most commonly used in conversation and casual writing.

PRACTICE QUESTIONS

Choose the word that BEST completes the sentence.

7. Her love _____ blueberry muffins kept her coming back to the bakery every week.

    A) to

    B) with

    C) of

    D) about

8. Christine left her house early on Monday morning, _____ she was still late for work.

    A) but

    B) and

    C) for

    D) or

Answer Key

1. **C)** *Minnesota* and *August* are proper nouns, and *coat* and *gloves* are common nouns. *I* is a pronoun, and *warm* is an adjective that modifies *coat*.

2. **B)** "The members of the band" is plural, so the plural pronoun *their* should be used instead of the singular *her*.

3. **A)** Choice A should read "The brother and sister run very fast." When the subject contains two or more nouns connected by *and*, the subject is plural and requires a plural verb.

4. **C)** Choice C should read "Johnny will go to the movies after he cleans the kitchen." It does not make sense to say that Johnny does something in the past ("went to the movies") after doing something in the present ("after he cleans").

5. **A)** *New* modifies the noun *chef*, and *boiling* modifies the noun *soup*. *Carefully* is an adverb modifying the verb *stirred*. *Lowered* is a verb, and *heat* is a noun.

6. **D)** Choice D should read "Of the four speeches, Jerry's was the longest." The word *long* has only one syllable, so it should be modified with the suffix *–est*, not the word *most*.

7. **C)** The correct preposition is *of*.

8. **A)** In this sentence, the conjunction joins together two contrasting ideas, so the correct answer is *but*.

12 | Sentence Structure

Phrases

To understand what a phrase is, you have to know about subjects and predicates. The **subject** is what the sentence is about; the **predicate** contains the verb and its modifiers.

> The nurse at the front desk will answer any questions you have.

The subject is "The nurse at the front desk," and the predicate is "will answer any questions you have."

A **phrase** is a group of words that communicates only part of an idea because it lacks either a subject or a predicate. Phrases are categorized based on the main word in the phrase. A **prepositional phrase** begins with a preposition and ends with an object of the preposition, a **verb phrase** is composed of the main verb along with any helping verbs, and a **noun phrase** consists of a noun and its modifiers.

> Prepositional phrase: The dog is hiding <u>under the porch</u>.
> Verb phrase: The chef <u>wanted to cook</u> a different dish.
> Noun phrase: <u>The big red barn</u> rests beside <u>the vacant chicken house</u>.

PRACTICE QUESTION

1. Identify the type of phrase underlined in the following sentence.

   The new patient was assigned to the nurse <u>with the most experience</u>.

   A) prepositional phrase

   B) noun phrase

   C) verb phrase

   D) verbal phrase

Clauses

Clauses contain both a subject and a predicate. They can be either independent or dependent. An **independent** (or main) **clause** can stand alone as its own sentence.

> The dog ate her homework.

Dependent (or subordinate) clauses cannot stand alone as their own sentences. They start with a subordinating conjunction, relative pronoun, or relative adjective, which makes them sound incomplete.

> <u>Because</u> the dog ate her homework

A sentence can be classified as simple, compound, complex, or compound-complex based on the type and number of clauses it has.

TABLE 12.1. Types of Clauses

SENTENCE TYPE	NUMBER OF INDEPENDENT CLAUSES	NUMBER OF DEPENDENT CLAUSES
Simple	1	0
Compound	2 or more	0
Complex	1	1 or more
Compound-complex	2 or more	1 or more

💡 **HELPFUL HINT**

On the test you will have to both identify and construct different kinds of sentences.

A **simple sentence** consists of one independent clause. Because there are no dependent clauses in a simple sentence, it can be a two-word sentence, with one word being the subject and the other word being the verb, such as *I ran*. However, a simple sentence can also contain prepositions, adjectives, and adverbs. Even though these additions can extend the length of a simple sentence, that sentence is still considered a simple sentence as long as it does not contain any dependent clauses.

> Simple: San Francisco in the springtime is one of my favorite places to visit.

Although the sentence is lengthy, it is simple because it contains only one subject and one verb (*San Francisco* and *is*), modified by additional phrases.

Compound sentences have two or more independent clauses and no dependent clauses. Usually, a comma and a coordinating conjunction (the FANBOYS: For, And, Nor, But, Or, Yet, and So) join the independent clauses, though semicolons can be used as well.

> Compound: The game was canceled, but we will still practice on Saturday.

This sentence is made up of two independent clauses joined by a conjunction (*but*), so it is compound.

Complex sentences have one independent clause and at least one dependent clause. The two clauses are joined by a subordinating conjunction.

> Complex: I love listening to the radio in the car
> because I can sing along.

The sentence has one independent clause ("I love listening to the radio in the car") and one dependent ("because I can sing along"), so it is complex.

Compound-complex sentences have two or more independent clauses and at least one dependent clause. Compound-complex sentences have both a coordinating and a subordinating conjunction.

> Complex: I wanted to get a dog, but I have a fish because my
> roommate is allergic to pet dander.

This sentence has three clauses: two independent ("I wanted to get a dog" and "I have a fish") and one dependent ("because my roommate is allergic to pet dander"), so it is compound-complex.

PRACTICE QUESTIONS

2. Which of the following choices is a simple sentence?

    A) Elsa drove, while Erica navigated.

    B) Betty ordered a fruit salad, and Sue ordered eggs.

    C) Because she was late, Jenny ran down the hall.

    D) John ate breakfast with his mother, brother, and father.

3. Which of the following sentences is a compound-complex sentence?

    A) While they were at the game, Anne cheered for the home team, but Harvey rooted for the underdogs.

    B) The rain flooded all of the driveway, some of the yard, and even part of the sidewalk across the street.

    C) After everyone finished the test, Mr. Brown passed a bowl of candy around the classroom.

    D) All the flowers in the front yard are in bloom, and the trees around the house are lush and green.

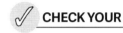

CHECK YOUR UNDERSTANDING

Can you write a simple, compound, complex, and compound-complex sentence using the same independent clause?

Punctuation

The basic rules for using the major punctuation marks are given in Table 12.2.

→
CONTINUE

TABLE 12.2. How to Use Punctuation

PUNCTUATION	USED FOR	EXAMPLE
Period	ending sentences	Periods go at the end of complete sentences.
Question mark	ending questions	What's the best way to end a sentence?
Exclamation point	ending sentences that show extreme emotion	I'll never understand how to use commas!
Comma	joining two independent clauses (always with a coordinating conjunction)	Commas can be used to join clauses, but they must always be followed by a coordinating conjunction.
	setting apart introductory and nonessential words and phrases	Commas, when used properly, set apart extra information in a sentence.
	separating items in a list	My favorite punctuation marks include the colon, semicolon, and period.
Semicolon	joining together two independent clauses (never used with a conjunction)	I love exclamation points; they make sentences seem so exciting!
Colon	introducing a list, explanation, or definition	When I see a colon, I know what to expect: more information.
Apostrophe	forming contractions	It's amazing how many people can't use apostrophes correctly.
	showing possession	Parentheses are my sister's favorite punctuation; she finds commas' rules confusing.
Quotation marks	indicating a direct quote	I said to her, "Tell me more about parentheses."

PRACTICE QUESTIONS

4. Which of the following sentences contains an error in punctuation?

   A) I love apple pie! John exclaimed with a smile.

   B) Jennifer loves Adam's new haircut.

   C) Billy went to the store; he bought bread, milk, and cheese.

   D) Alexandra hates raisins, but she loves chocolate chips.

5. Which punctuation mark correctly completes the sentence?

> Sam, why don't you come with us for dinner_

A) .

B) ;

C) ?

D) :

Capitalization

Capitalization questions on the TEAS will ask you to spot errors in capitalization within a phrase or sentence. Below are the most important rules for capitalization you are likely to see on the test.

The first word of a sentence is always capitalized.

> We will be having dinner at a new restaurant tonight.

The first letter of a proper noun is always capitalized.

> We're going to Chicago on Wednesday.

Titles are capitalized if they precede the name they modify.

> Kamala Harris, the vice president, met with President Biden.

Months are capitalized, but not the names of the seasons.

> Snow fell in March even though winter was over.

The names of major holidays should be capitalized. The word *day* is only capitalized if it is part of the holiday's name.

> We always go to a parade on Memorial Day,
> but Christmas day we stay home.

The names of specific places should always be capitalized. General location terms are not capitalized.

> We're going to San Francisco next weekend so I can see the ocean.

Titles for relatives should be capitalized when they precede a name, but not when they stand alone.

> Fred, my uncle, will make fried chicken, and Aunt Kiki is going to
> make spaghetti.

PRACTICE QUESTION

6. Which of the following sentences contains an error in capitalization?

A) My two brothers are going to New Orleans for Mardi Gras.

B) On Friday we voted to elect a new class president.

C) Janet wants to go to Mexico this Spring.

D) Peter complimented the chef on his cooking.

Homophones and Spelling

The TEAS will include questions that ask you to choose between **homophones**, words that are pronounced the same but have different meanings. *Bawl* and *ball*, for example, are homophones: they sound the same, but the first means "to cry," and the second is a round toy.

Common homophones include:

- bare/bear
- brake/break
- die/dye
- effect/affect
- flour/flower
- heal/heel
- insure/ensure
- morning/mourning
- peace/piece
- poor/pour
- principal/principle
- sole/soul
- stair/stare
- suite/sweet
- their/there/they're
- wear/where

You will also be tested on spelling, so it is good to familiarize yourself with commonly misspelled words and special spelling rules. The test questions will ask you to either find a misspelled word in a sentence or identify words that don't follow standard spelling rules.

Double a final consonant when adding suffixes if the consonant is preceded by a single vowel.

run → running
admit → admittance

Drop the final vowel when adding a suffix.

> sue → suing
> observe → observance

Change the final *y* to an *i* when adding a suffix.

> lazy → laziest
> tidy → tidily

Regular nouns are made plural by adding *s*. Irregular nouns can follow many different rules for pluralization, which are summarized in the table below.

TABLE 12.3. Irregular Plural Nouns

ENDS WITH ...	MAKE IT PLURAL BY ...	EXAMPLE
y	changing *y* to *i* and adding *–es*	baby → babies
f	changing *f* to *v* and adding *–es*	leaf → leaves
fe	changing *f* to *v* and adding *–s*	knife → knives
o	adding *–es*	potato → potatoes
us	changing *–us* to *–i*	nucleus → nuclei

Always the same	Doesn't follow the rules
sheep deer fish moose pants binoculars scissors	man → men child → children person → people tooth → teeth goose → geese mouse → mice ox → oxen

Commonly Misspelled Words

- accommodate
- across
- argument
- believe
- committee
- completely

- conscious
- discipline
- experience
- foreign
- government
- guarantee
- height
- immediately
- intelligence
- judgment
- knowledge
- license
- lightning
- lose
- maneuver
- misspell
- noticeable
- occasionally
- occurred
- opinion
- personnel
- piece
- possession
- receive
- separate
- successful
- technique
- tendency
- unanimous
- until
- usually
- vacuum
- whether
- which

Some words are similar in meaning but are not synonyms. However, they are commonly confused in writing and speech. A hallmark of good writing is the proper use of these words.

TABLE 12.4. Commonly Confused Words

CONFUSED WORDS	DEFINITION
Amount	describes a noncountable quantity (*an unknown amount of jewelry was stolen*)
Number	describes a countable quantity (*an unknown number of necklaces was stolen*)
Bring	toward the speaker (*bring to me*)
Take	away from the speaker (*take away from me*)
Farther	a measurable distance (*the house farther up the road*)
Further	more or greater (*explain further what you mean*)
Fewer	a smaller amount of something plural (*fewer chairs*)
Less	a smaller amount of something that cannot be counted (*less water*)
Lose	to fail to win; to not be able to find something (*to lose a game; to lose one's keys*)
Loose	relaxed; not firmly in place (*my pants are loose*)

PRACTICE QUESTIONS

7. Which of the following sentences contains a spelling error?

    A) It was unusually warm that winter, so we didn't need to use our fireplace.

    B) Our garden includes tomatos, squash, and carrots.

    C) The local zoo will be opening a new exhibit that includes African elephants.

    D) My sister is learning to speak a foreign language so she can travel abroad.

8. Which of the following words correctly completes the sentence?

    The nurse has three _____ to see before lunch.

    A) patents

    B) patience

    C) patients

    D) patient's

9. Which of the following words correctly completes the sentence?

    Without a proper chain of evidence, we could _____ the case.

    A) lose

    B) loose

    C) loss

    D) loses

10. Which of the following words correctly completes the sentence?

There were _____ cars this morning in the parking lot than usual.

A) less

B) fewer

C) several

D) enough

Answer Key

1. **A)** The underlined section of the sentence is a prepositional phrase beginning with the preposition *with*.

2. **D)** Choice D contains one independent clause with one subject and one verb. Choices A and C are complex sentences because they each contain both a dependent and independent clause. Choice B contains two independent clauses joined by a conjunction and is therefore a compound sentence.

3. **A)** Choice A is a compound-complex sentence because it contains two independent clauses and one dependent clause. Despite its length, choice B is a simple sentence because it contains only one independent clause. Choice C is a complex sentence because it contains one dependent clause and one independent clause. Choice D is a compound sentence; it contains two independent clauses.

4. **A)** Choice A should use quotation marks to set off a direct quote: *"I love apple pie!" John exclaimed with a smile.*

5. **C)** The sentence is a question, so it should end with a question mark.

6. **C)** *Spring* is the name of a season and should not be capitalized.

7. **B)** *Tomatos* should be spelled *tomatoes*.

8. **C)** *Patients* is the correct spelling and the correct homophone. A *patent* is proof that someone owns the rights to an invention or idea. *Patience* is the ability to avoid getting upset in negative situations. *Patient's*, which contains an apostrophe, is the singular possessive form of *patient*.

9. **A)** To *lose* is to fail to win. *Loose* means "not firmly in place." *Loss* is a noun, and *loses* is incorrectly conjugated; neither choice makes sense in context.

10. **B)** *Fewer* is used to indicate a smaller amount of something plural (in this case, *cars*). *Less* is used to indicate a smaller amount of something that cannot be counted (for instance, water or air). *Several* and *enough* do not make sense in context.

13 | Writing

The Writing Process

A writer's task is to convey information and meaning accurately and effectively. To do so, writers develop sentences, paragraphs, and whole texts.

The **writing process** typically involves the following steps:

- **prewriting** (planning, mapping, or brainstorming)
- **drafting** (writing and constructing)
- **revising** (moving, cutting, replacing, and adding)
- **editing** (checking grammar and punctuation)
- **proofreading** (checking the final draft for typos)

Throughout the writing process, it is essential that a writer ensure unity in a text. **Unity** demands that the details included in a sentence, paragraph, or text share a main idea.

For example, all ideas within a paragraph must support the main idea that is expressed in the paragraph's topic sentence (often the first sentence of the paragraph). Similarly, the thesis statement for a larger work will unify ideas across paragraphs and the full text.

There are many kinds of details that writers can use to support their main idea. Writing is more interesting and convincing when writers use a variety of types of details. Many writers refer to the acronym **RENNS** to recall these various types:

- Reasons
- Examples
- Names
- Numbers
- Senses

The logical progression of words, sentences, and paragraphs makes a piece of writing coherent. To assist with coherence, writers employ **transitional expressions**, some of which are listed in Table 13.1.

TABLE 13.1. Transitional Expressions	
MEANING	**EXPRESSIONS**
Addition	and, furthermore, moreover, too, also, in addition, next, besides, first, second
Contrast	although, in contrast, but, conversely, nevertheless, however, on the contrary, on the other hand
Time	later, earlier, when, while, soon, thereafter, meanwhile, whenever, during, now, until now, subsequently
Location	nearby, adjacent to, beyond, above, below
Comparison	similarly, in the same manner, in like manner, likewise
Cause	because, since, on account of, for that reason
Illustration	specifically, for instance, for example
Effect	therefore, consequently, accordingly, as a result
Summation	in summary, in brief, to sum up
Conclusion	in conclusion, finally
Referring back to an object or idea	this, that, these, those (To avoid a pronoun reference error, the pronoun reference must be clear and near the antecedent.)
To replace a noun	Use personal pronouns for coherence to avoid unnecessary redundancies.

Using different types of sentences also helps maintain the reader's interest. Writers should begin sentences differently, making some sentences long and some sentences short. Writers should use simple sentences and complex sentences that have complex ideas in them.

Readers appreciate variety, but the priority is for sentences to make sense. It's better to have clear and simple writing that a reader can understand than to have complex, confusing syntax that does not clearly express the idea.

After completing the writing task, the writer should look it over and checking for spelling and grammar mistakes that may interfere with a reader's understanding.

PRACTICE QUESTION

1. When should the drafting process begin?
   A) after revisions
   B) following proofreading
   C) before prewriting
   D) after prewriting

Organizing Writing

Almost all writing begins with an **introduction**, which sets the tone, topic, direction, style, and mood for the writing that is to follow. Most importantly, the introduction provides the first impression of the writer to the reader. Thus, writers must create introductions that are engaging and appropriate for their audience.

Body paragraphs provide information to support a writer's argument or point of view. Most paragraphs are centered around a **topic sentence**, a sentence that explains the topic of the paragraph. The topic sentence usually appears as the first sentence of a paragraph.

Paragraphs should be structurally consistent, beginning with a topic sentence to introduce the main idea, followed by supporting ideas and examples. No extra ideas unrelated to the paragraph's focus should appear. Transition words and phrases should connect body paragraphs and improve the flow and readability of a piece of writing.

A **conclusion** leaves the reader with a sense of closure by reiterating the author's thesis and sometimes even providing a summary of the main points. Between the introduction and the conclusion, a writer may develop a text using different organizational patterns.

A particularly useful tool for organizing ideas is the outline. An **outline** is an overall map of the content of a text; it may be informal or formal, phrasal, or clausal.

A formal outline for a written essay should include the following elements: an introduction, a thesis statement, main points in grammatically similar structure, subpoints in grammatically similar structure, active voice, action verbs, a restatement of the thesis, and a conclusion.

PRACTICE QUESTION

2. How should a writer begin when working on well-organized writing?

   A) develop a formal outline

   B) start by writing the conclusion

   C) write the topic sentence for each paragraph

   D) make a list of transition phrases to be used

Revising Informal and Formal Language

Writers tailor language to appeal to the intended audience, so the reader can determine from the language who the author is speaking to. **Formal writing** is used in business and academic settings and can make the author seem more credible. Characteristics of a formal style include

- third-person perspective (avoiding the use of *I* or *you*);

- no slang or cliches;

- following a clear structure (an introduction, a body, and a conclusion, for example);
- technically correct grammar and sentence structure;
- objective language.

Informal writing is used to appeal to readers in a more casual setting, such as a magazine or blog. Using an informal style may make the author seem less credible, but it can help create an emotional connection with the audience. Characteristics of informal writing include

- first or second person perspective (*I* or *you*, for example);
- slang or casual language;
- following an unusual or flexible structure;
- bending the rules of grammar;
- appealing to the audience's emotions.

PRACTICE QUESTION

Answer the question based on the passage below.

> What do you do with plastic bottles? Do you throw them away, or do you recycle or reuse them? As landfills continue to fill up, there will eventually be no place to put garbage. If you recycle or reuse bottles, you will help reduce waste.

3. How could this passage be revised to make it more formal?
   A) change the writing to third person from direct address
   B) replace "landfills" with "trash dumps"
   C) replace "garbage" with "trash"
   D) rewrite the passage in the past tense

Avoiding Bias

A writer should account for **culturally diverse language** and avoid bias in writing. The pronouns *he*, *him*, and *his* are not considered gender neutral. Writing should be revised to avoid this bias:

Wrong: Each student should study for his exam.

Correct: All students should study for their exams.

Many common nouns can be rewritten to be gender neutral:

congressman → congressperson

male nurse → nurse

mailman → postal carrier

Person-first language is generally preferred when discussing health conditions or disabilities. This humanizes the subject. Revise for person-first language to avoid stereotypes and bias:

Wrong: a patient suffering from diabetes; a diabetic patient

Correct: a patient who has diabetes; a patient with diabetes

PRACTICE QUESTION

4. Which of the following sentences should be revised to avoid bias?

    A) Physicians typically study for many years.

    B) I avoid man-made chemicals, so I eat organic food.

    C) The police officer questioned the suspect.

    D) Nurses should listen to patients' concerns.

Answer Key

1. **D)** The drafting process begins after the prewriting process.

2. **A)** A formal outline helps writers organize their thoughts by mapping out the text before writing it. Well-organized writing starts with an outline.

3. **A)** The informal tone and direct address of this passage suggest that the author is writing for a general audience. Rewriting it in the third person would make it more formal.

4. **B)** "Man-made" should be revised. It could be replaced with words like "synthetic" or "artificial": "I avoid artificial chemicals, so I eat organic food."

Reading

Directions: Read the question, passage, or figure carefully, and choose the best answer.

Questions 1 – 4 are based on the following passage.

In recent decades, jazz has been associated with New Orleans and festivals like Mardi Gras, but in the 1920s jazz was a booming trend whose influence reached into many aspects of American culture. In fact, the years between World War I and the Great Depression were known as the Jazz Age, a term coined by F. Scott Fitzgerald in his famous novel *The Great Gatsby*. Sometimes also called the Roaring Twenties, this time period saw major urban centers experience new economic, cultural, and artistic vitality. In the United States, musicians flocked to cities like New York and Chicago, which would become famous hubs for jazz musicians. Ella Fitzgerald, for example, moved from Virginia to New York City to begin her much-lauded singing career, and jazz pioneer Louis Armstrong got his big break in Chicago.

Jazz music was played by and for a more expressive and freer populace than the United States had previously seen. Women gained the right to vote and were openly seen drinking and wearing revealing clothing. This period marked the emergence of the flapper, a woman determined to make a statement about her new role in society. Jazz music also provided the soundtrack for the explosion of African American art and culture now known as the Harlem Renaissance. In addition to Fitzgerald and Armstrong, numerous musicians, including Duke Ellington, Fats Waller, and Bessie Smith, promoted their distinctive and complex music as an integral part of the emerging African American culture.

1. Which of the following is the author's main purpose for writing this passage?

   A) to explain the role jazz musicians played in the Harlem Renaissance

   B) to inform the reader about the many important musicians playing jazz in the 1920s

   C) to discuss how jazz influenced important cultural movements in the 1920s

   D) to provide a history of jazz music in the twentieth century

2. The sentence below appears in the second paragraph of the passage.

   Jazz music also provided the soundtrack for the explosion of African American art and culture now known as the Harlem Renaissance.

   This sentence is BEST described as which of the following?

   A) theme

   B) topic

   C) main idea

   D) supporting idea

CONTINUE

3. The passage demonstrates which of the following types of writing?

   A) technical

   B) expository

   C) persuasive

   D) narrative

4. Which of the following conclusions may be drawn directly from the second paragraph of the passage?

   A) Jazz music was important to minority groups struggling for social equality in the 1920s.

   B) Duke Ellington, Fats Waller, and Bessie Smith were the most important jazz musicians of the Harlem Renaissance.

   C) Women were able to gain the right to vote with the help of jazz musicians.

   D) Duke Ellington, Fats Waller, and Bessie Smith all supported women's right to vote.

Questions 5 – 8 are based on the passage below.

Popcorn is often associated with fun and festivities, both in and out of the home. It's eaten in theaters, usually after being salted and smothered in butter, and in homes, fresh from the microwave. But popcorn isn't just for fun—it's also a multimillion-dollar industry with a long and fascinating history.

While popcorn might seem like a modern invention, its history actually dates back thousands of years, making it one of the oldest snack foods enjoyed around the world. Popping is believed by food historians to be one of the earliest uses of cultivated corn. In 1948, Herbert Dick and Earle Smith discovered old popcorn dating back 4,000 years in the New Mexico Bat Cave. For the Aztec Indians that called the caves home, popcorn (or *momochitl*) played an important role in society, both as a food staple and in ceremonies. The Aztecs cooked popcorn by heating sand in a fire; when it was heated, kernels were added and would pop when exposed to the heat of the sand.

The American love affair with popcorn began in 1912, when popcorn was first sold in theaters. The popcorn industry flourished during the Great Depression by advertising popcorn as a wholesome and economical food. Selling for five to ten cents a bag, it was a luxury that the downtrodden could afford. With the introduction of mobile popcorn

machines at the World's Columbian Exposition in the late 1800s, popcorn moved from the theater into fairs and parks. Popcorn continued to rule the snack food kingdom until the rise in popularity of home televisions during the 1950s.

The popcorn industry reacted to its decline in sales quickly by introducing pre-popped and un-popped popcorn for home consumption. However, it wasn't until microwave popcorn became commercially available in 1981 that at-home popcorn consumption began to grow exponentially. With the wide availability of microwaves in the United States, popcorn also began popping up in offices and hotel rooms. The home still remains the most popular popcorn eating spot, though: Today, 70 percent of the 16 billion quarts of popcorn consumed annually in the United States is eaten at home.

5. The author's description of the growth of the popcorn industry demonstrates which of the following types of text structure?

   A) cause-effect

   B) comparison-contrast

   C) chronological

   D) problem-solution

6. Which of the following conclusions may be drawn directly from the third paragraph of the passage?

   A) People ate less popcorn in the 1950s than in previous decades because they went to the movies less.

   B) Without mobile popcorn machines, people would not have been able to eat popcorn during the Great Depression.

   C) People enjoyed popcorn during the Great Depression because it was a luxury food.

   D) During the 1800s, people began abandoning theaters to go to fairs and festivals.

7. Which of the following is the author's main purpose for writing this passage?

   A) to explain how microwaves affected the popcorn industry

   B) to show that popcorn is older than many people realize

   C) to illustrate the history of popcorn from ancient cultures to modern times

   D) to demonstrate the importance of popcorn in various cultures

8. Based on the passage, which of the following is the most likely inference?

   A) Popcorn tastes better when it is cooked on heated sand.

   B) The popcorn industry will continue to thrive in the United States.

   C) If movie theaters go out of business, the popcorn industry will also fail.

   D) Archaeologists would likely find other examples of ancient cultures eating popcorn if they looked hard enough.

Questions 9 and 10 are based on the passage below.

Mason was one of those guys who just always seemed at home. Stick him on a bus, and he'd make three new friends; when he joined a team, it was only a matter of time before he was elected captain. This particular skill rested almost entirely in his eyes. These brown orbs seemed lit from within, and when Mason focused that fire, it was impossible not to feel its warmth. People sought out Mason for the feeling of comfort he so easily created, and anyone with a good joke would want to tell it to Mason. His laughter started with a spark in his eyes that traveled down to create his wide, open smile.

9. Based on a prior knowledge of literature, the reader can infer that this passage was taken from which of the following?

   A) a short-story collection

   B) a science magazine

   C) an academic journal

   D) a history textbook

10. Which of the following is a logical conclusion that can be drawn from this description?

    A) Mason wishes people would tell him more jokes.

    B) Mason is very good at sports.

    C) Mason does not like when strangers approach him.

    D) Mason has many friends.

Questions 11 and 12 are based on the following memo.

MEMO

From: Human Resource Department

To: Department Leaders

Date: December 6, 2018

Subject: Personal Use of Computers

Management has been conducting standard monitoring of computer usage, and we are dismayed at the amount of personal use occurring during business hours. Employee computers are available for the sole purpose of completing company business and for nothing else. These rules must be respected. If employees are found to be using computers for personal use during work hours, disciplinary action will be taken. Personal use should occur in emergency situations only, and in these cases, use should be limited to 30 minutes. Please communicate these requirements to all personnel in your department.

11. Which of the following is the main purpose of this email?

    A) to notify employees that their computer use is being monitored

    B) to inform a group of employees about disciplinary action that has been taken

    C) to provide information about the computer usage policy to department leaders

    D) to explain in which emergency situations it is appropriate for employees to use computers

12. Which of the following inferences may be logically drawn from the memo?

    A) Department leaders will be punished if employees are found to be using computers inappropriately.

    B) Employees will likely leave the company rather than stop using their computers for personal business.

    C) Management will allow some flexibility in the rules for computer use among department leaders.

    D) Management will not hesitate to initiate disciplinary action against employees who use computers inappropriately.

Questions 13 – 15 are based on the following passage.

It could be said that the great battle between the North and South we call the Civil War was a battle for individual identity. The states of the South had their own culture, one based on farming, independence, and the rights of both man and state to determine their own paths. Similarly, the North had forged its own identity as a center of centralized commerce and manufacturing. This clash of lifestyles was bound to create tension, and this tension was bound to lead to war. But people who try to sell you this narrative are wrong. The Civil War was not a battle of cultural identities—it was a battle about slavery. All other explanations for the war are either a direct consequence of the South's desire for wealth at the expense of her fellow man or a fanciful invention to cover up this sad portion of our nation's history. And it cannot be denied that this time in our past was very sad indeed.

13. Which of the following describes this type of writing?

    A) technical

    B) expository

    C) persuasive

    D) narrative

14. Which of the following is a likely motive of the author?

    A) to convince readers that slavery was the main cause of the Civil War

    B) to illustrate the cultural differences between the North and the South before the Civil War

    C) to persuade readers that the North deserved to win the Civil War

    D) to demonstrate that the history of the Civil War is too complicated to be understood clearly

15. Which of the following statements BEST describes the author's point of view?

    A) The Civil War was the result of cultural differences between the North and South.

    B) The Civil War was caused by the South's reliance on slave labor.

    C) The North's use of commerce and manufacturing allowed them to win the war.

    D) The South's belief in the rights of man and state cost them the war.

Questions 16 and 17 are based on the following passage.

Patients are to arrive at the hospital two hours before the scheduled start time for their surgery. All surgery patients must check in at the Hospital Admissions Desk before proceeding to the Third-Floor Surgery Admissions Desk. The admitting nurse will ensure that all required paperwork has been completed before the patient is taken to the Surgery Holding Room. Once admitted to the Holding Room, the patient will need permission from the head nurse to leave and reenter. One family member or friend may accompany the patient in the Holding Room. All other family and friends will be asked to remain in the Third-Floor Waiting Area.

16. Which of the following is the first place a patient entering the hospital would visit?

    A) Surgery Admissions Desk

    B) Hospital Admissions Desk

    C) Surgery Holding Room

    D) Third-Floor Waiting Area

17. A patient who has checked in at the Surgery Admissions Desk would go to which location next?

    A) Surgery Admissions Desk

    B) Hospital Admissions Desk

    C Surgery Holding Room

    D) Third-Floor Waiting Area

18. Which of the following is a primary source for an article on the Battle of Gettysburg?

    A) a letter written by a local farmer who witnessed the battle

    B) a documentary about the battle produced by a local TV station

    C) a novelization of the battle written by the great-grandson of a Union soldier

    D) a history textbook for a college-level course in American history

Question 19 is based on the following lists.

Tree Species by Ecosystem

Tropical Rain Forest: mahogany, Brazil nut, rubber tree, tualang, strangler figs

Tropical Dry Forest: palu, Ceylon ebony, governor's plum

Temperate Deciduous Forest: oak, maple, beech, elm, magnolia, sweet gum

Temperate Coniferous Forest: cedar, cypress, juniper, pine, spruce, redwood

19. According to the lists above, beech trees are found in which ecosystem?

   A) tropical rain forest

   B) tropical dry forest

   C) temperate deciduous forest

   D) temperate coniferous forest

20. Which of the following sentences indicates the end of a sequence?

   A) Unfortunately, the stock did not perform as well as we had hoped.

   B) The next day, we were able to find a band we liked that also fit our budget.

   C) Overall, my friends and I found the experience rewarding.

   D) Before we go to the restaurant, let's look at the menu.

21. The index below is from a psychology textbook.

Memory, types, 315 – 347
    autobiographical, 326
    explicit, 316 – 320
    implicit, 319 – 325
    long-term, 333 – 342
    short-term, 340 – 346

   Which of the following pages should a reader check first for information on short-term memory?

   A) 316

   B) 319

   C) 333

   D) 340

The next two questions are based on the figure below.

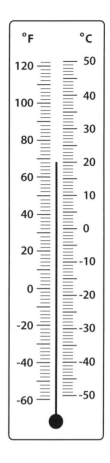

22. If the thermometer indicated a temperature of −40°F, what would the temperature be in degrees Celsius?

   A) −40°C

   B) −34°C

   C) −6°C

   D) 85°C

23. If the reading on the thermometer dropped 10°C, what would the temperature be in degrees Fahrenheit?

   A) 50°F

   B) 60°F

   C) 78°F

   D) 76°F

CONTINUE

The next three questions are based on the figure showing the inventory at Gigi's Diner below.

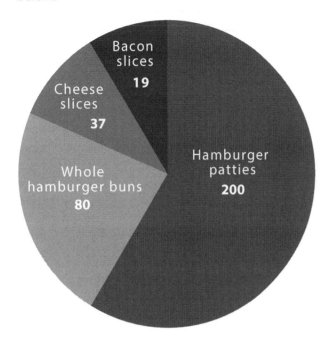

24. Which food does Gigi's have the least of?

    A) bacon slices

    B) cheese slices

    C) hamburger buns

    D) hamburger patties

25. According to the graph, how many more hamburger buns does Gigi's need in order to make 200 hamburgers?

    A) 120

    B) 161

    C) 181

    D) 200

26. How many hamburgers could Gigi's make if each burger includes one bacon slice and two cheese slices?

    A) 18

    B) 19

    C) 39

    D) 80

27. Which of the following BEST defines the word *eloquent* as used in the sentence that follows?

The president's speech was eloquent and touched many voters with its wit and flair.

    A) long-winded

    B) dispassionate

    C) loud

    D) well-spoken

Questions 28 – 30 are based on the passage below.

From the outside, your ears may look like floppy satellite dishes that are perpetually begging you to insert the latest wireless earphones. But did you know that your ears are more than just auditory conduits for the latest tunes? When you move past these whirlpools of flesh and cartilage and into the narrow catacombs of your inner ear, you enter an entirely different physiological realm. The ear has a secret secondary job: balance.

The labyrinth of your inner ear—literally called the bony labyrinth—is composed of a series of waxy canals and fluid-filled ducts. In addition to the cochlea, which is responsible for hearing, you have five balance receptors. Two receptors detect linear motion: one for up-and-down movement and the other for forward-and-backward or side-to-side movements. The other three receptors—the semicircular canals—work together to detect head rotation. The semicircular canals are at right angles to each other, replicating the three dimensions of the world around us. They contain a special fluid called endolymph, which "sloshes" with the movement of your head, stimulating tiny hairlike structures that then send signals to your brain about the direction you are moving—or whether you are still. So think twice before you inundate your dual-purpose ears with the deafening reverberations of the top forty—you might be throwing your whole world off balance.

28. Readers can infer from the passage that the author is trying to

    A) inform and persuade.

    B) inform and entertain.

    C) warn and persuade.

    D) amuse and entertain.

29. Why does the author use the hyphenated word *dual-purpose* in the last sentence?

    A) to show that our ears have two jobs: hearing and helping us keep our balance

    B) to show that we have two ears and two eyes, but only one nose

    C) to jokingly refer to a play on words: "you might be throwing your whole world off balance"

    D) to rhyme with the phrase "cruel chirp hiss"

30. According to the passage, two out of five "receptors" in the ear "detect linear motion." What do the other three receptors do?

    A) They allow us to hear sounds.

    B) They form a bony labyrinth.

    C) They detect head rotation.

    D) They tell us when music is too noisy.

Questions 31 and 32 are based on the passage below.

Most people think of respiration as the mechanical exchange of air between human lungs and the environment. They think about oxygen filling up the tiny air sacs in the lungs. They think about how this process feeds the capillaries surrounding the air sacs, which then infuse the bloodstream with the oxygen it needs. They may even think about how carbon dioxide is exhaled from the lungs back into the environment. But this process—known as external respiration—is just one form of respiration that occurs in the human body. Did you know there are actually two types of respiration in humans? The second form of respiration is equally important; it is known as internal, or cellular, respiration.

Whereas external respiration centers on an exchange between the lungs and the environment, internal respiration centers on a molecular exchange between cells and capillaries. All organs inside the human body rely on cellular respiration to function properly. Cells within the organs are surrounded by thousands of tiny capillaries that act as channels for the exchange of gases. Oxygen is carried through these microscopic blood vessels, moving from red blood cells to the surrounding tissue. Additionally, built-up carbon dioxide in the tissues flows through the capillaries back to the lungs. This second form of respiration may be invisible to the human eye, but it is crucial for the maintenance of human life.

31. Which of the following statements can the reader infer from the passage?

    A) The author believes that most people know what capillaries are.

    B) The idea that the human lungs contain tiny air sacs is a myth.

    C) The term "external respiration" does not accurately describe breathing.

    D) The author believes that most people have never heard of internal respiration.

32. What is the author's primary purpose in writing this essay?

    A) to inform readers about external and internal respiration

    B) to advise readers about ways to treat patients with lung disease

    C) to prove that most people are ignorant about internal respiration

    D) to persuade readers to take better care of their lungs and other organs

33. A student wants to look online to find unbiased information about organic foods. Analyze the following websites and their taglines to determine which site he should use.

    A) www.dangerinthegrocerystore.com; "The truth about the toxic chemicals in your produce."

    B) www.growbetter.com; "Your one-stop shop for agricultural pesticides and fertilizers."

    C) www.betterfood.org; "A nonprofit that provides nutritional support to needy families."

    D) www.foodandnutrition.gov; "An official site of the United States Surgeon General."

34. The table of contents following is from an American history textbook.

Chapter 2: Early American History

    1. Early Settlement

        A. Plymouth

        B. Jamestown

    2. The American Revolution

        A. American Victories

        B. British Victories

3. A New Century
    A. The Constitutional Convention
    B. The Ratification Years

Which of the following lists includes only subheadings?

A) Plymouth, Jamestown, British Victories, and A New Century

B) American Victories, British Victories, A New Century, and The Ratification Years

C) American Victories, British Victories, The Constitutional Convention, and The Ratification Years

D) Early Settlement, The American Revolution, A New Century, and The Ratification Years

35. The directions below are from a plumbing manual.

When connecting line A to port B, make sure that port C is **completely** closed. If port C is left open, fluid will leak as soon as line A is connected. Once line A and port B are **fully** connected, port C can be opened as needed.

The bold text in the directions indicates which of the following?

A) brand names

B) emphasis

C) commands

D) proper nouns

36. Read and follow the directions below.

1. You start with $20 in your wallet.
2. You spend $5 on lunch.
3. You receive $20 for mowing your neighbor's yard.
4. You spend $10 on a new shirt.
5. You receive $10 for driving a friend to work.
6. You spend $30 on fuel for your vehicle.

How much money do you have left?

A) $0

B) $5

C) $10

D) $20

37. After following the directions below, how much water is left?

1. You have 3 gallons of water.
2. You use 0.5 gallons to water your plant.
3. You use 1 gallon to refill your dog's water bowl.
4. You put 0.5 gallons in an ice tray to make ice cubes.

A) 0 gallons

B) 0.5 gallons

C) 1 gallon

D) 1.5 gallons

38. Which of the following BEST defines the underlined word in the sentence below?

Elaine was feeling lethargic after a poor night's sleep, but she still managed to get to work on time.

A) tired

B) confused

C) angry

D) rushed

39. The headings below are from an art history textbook.

Chapter 6: Art of the Middle Ages
I. The Stories Behind Famous Paintings
II. Notable Sculpting Techniques
III. Recipes for Common Dishes
IV. Textiles and Tapestries

Which of the following headings does NOT belong in the outline?

A) The Stories Behind Famous Paintings

B) Notable Sculpting Techniques

C) Recipes for Common Dishes

D) Textiles and Tapestries

40. Read and follow the directions below.

1. Start at the center of town.
2. Drive north 10 miles.
3. Turn left and drive west 5 miles.
4. Turn left and drive south 2 miles.
5. Turn right and drive west 1 mile.

Which of the following is now your distance from the center of town?

A) 12 miles north, 6 miles west

B) 8 miles north, 6 miles west

C) 12 miles north, 4 miles west

D) 8 miles north, 4 miles west

41. Which of the following BEST defines the underlined word in the sentence below?

Miguel was concerned that his <u>laceration</u> would need stitches.

A) deep cut

B) minor wound

C) broken bone

D) swollen joint

42. The table of contents below is from a travel guide.

Chapter 3: Planning Your Vacation

 1. Getting There

   A. Air Travel

   B. Traveling by Train

   C. _____

   D. Taking the Bus

 2. Accommodations

 3. Dining

Based on the pattern of the headings, which of the following is a reasonable heading to insert in the blank spot?

A) Choosing a Destination

B) Navigating the Airport

C) Finding a Hotel

D) Road Trips

43. Read and follow the directions below.

1. You start with one red marble and two green marbles in a pouch.
2. Remove one red marble.
3. Add one green marble.
4. Add one red marble.
5. Add one green marble.
6. Remove one red marble.
7. Remove one green marble.
8. Add three red marbles.
9. Add two green marbles.

How many red and green marbles are now in the pouch?

A) five red, three green

B) three red, five green

C) four red, four green

D) six red, two green

44. Read the passage, and answer the question that follows.

The couple's "plan" was little more than just a desire to travel. They showed up at the airport with no tickets, no itinerary, and no destination in mind.

The use of quotation marks signifies which of the following?

A) foreign phrases

B) emphasized words

C) dialogue

D) words used ironically

45. How could the passage be revised to make it more formal?

A) remove the phrase "little more than"

B) remove the quotation marks from *plan*

C) change *showed up* to *arrived*

D) change *with no* to *without any*

→
CONTINUE

Mathematics

Directions: Read the question carefully, and choose the best answer.

1. If a person reads 40 pages in 45 minutes, approximately how many minutes will it take her to read 265 pages?

   A) 202

   B) 236

   C) 265

   D) 298

2. If a student answers 42 out of 48 questions correctly on a quiz, what percentage of questions did she answer correctly?

   A) 82.5%

   B) 85%

   C) 87.5%

   D) 90%

3. What is 1230.932567 rounded to the nearest hundredth?

   A) 1200

   B) 1230

   C) 1230.93

   D) 1230.9326

4. Melissa is ordering fencing to enclose a square area of 5625 square feet. How many feet of fencing does she need?

   A) 75

   B) 150

   C) 300

   D) 5625

5. If a discount of 25% off the retail price of a desk saves Mark $45, what was the desk's original price?

   A) $135

   B) $160

   C) $180

   D) $210

6. What number is 5% of 2000?

   A) 50

   B) 100

   C) 150

   D) 200

7. Jane earns $15 per hour babysitting. If she starts with $275 in her bank account, which equation represents how many hours (h) she will have to babysit for her account to reach $400?

   A) $400 = 275 + 15h$

   B) $400 = 15h$

   C) $400 = \frac{15}{h} + 275$

   D) $400 = -275 - 15h$

8. A circular swimming pool has a circumference of 50 feet. Which of the following is the diameter of the pool in feet?

   A) $\frac{25}{\pi}$

   B) $\frac{50}{\pi}$

   C) 25π

   D) 50π

9. A bag contains twice as many red marbles as blue marbles, and the number of blue marbles is 88% of the number of green marbles. If g represents the number of green marbles, which of the following expressions represents the total number of marbles in the bag?

   A) $2.32g$

   B) $2.64g$

   C) $3.64g$

   D) $3.88g$

10. Which of the following is listed in order from least to greatest?

    A) $-0.95, 0, \frac{2}{5}, 0.35, \frac{3}{4}$

    B) $-1, -\frac{1}{10}, -0.11, \frac{5}{6}, 0.75$

    C) $-\frac{3}{4}, -0.2, 0, \frac{2}{3}, 0.55$

    D) $-1.1, -\frac{4}{5}, -0.13, 0.7, \frac{9}{11}$

11. Which inequality is equivalent to $\frac{2x+7}{9} < 2$?

    A) $3x < 7$

    B) $x > -3$

    C) $x < \frac{11}{2}$

    D) $2x > 1$

12. How much longer is line segment *MN* than line segment *KL*?

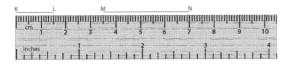

A) 2 mm

B) 15 mm

C) 20 mm

D) 55 mm

13. How much water is needed to fill 24 bottles that each hold 0.75 liters?

A) 6 L

B) 18 L

C) 24 L

D) 32 L

14. Which inequality is equivalent to $3x + 2 > 5$?

A) $x < 1$

B) $x > -1$

C) $x > 1$

D) $x > 3$

15. Michael is making cupcakes. He plans to give $\frac{1}{2}$ of the cupcakes to a friend and $\frac{1}{3}$ of the cupcakes to his coworkers. If he makes 48 cupcakes, how many will he have left over?

A) 8

B) 10

C) 16

D) 24

Use the chart below to answer questions 16 and 17.

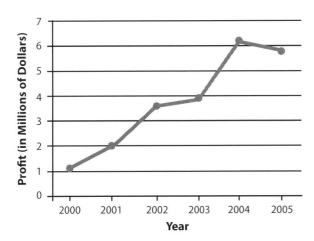

16. Referencing the line graph, approximately how much did profit increase from 2003 to 2004 in dollars?

A) 2.2 million

B) 3.2 million

C) 3.9 million

D) 6.2 million

17. Approximately how much more profit was earned in 2001 than in 2000?

A) 1.0 million

B) 2.2 million

C) 3.5 million

D) 6.1 million

18. Juan plans to spend 25% of his workday writing a report. If he is at work for 9 hours, how many hours will he spend writing the report?

A) 2.25

B) 2.50

C) 2.75

D) 4.00

19. Jessie leaves her home and rides her bike 12 miles south and then 16 miles east. She then takes the shortest possible route back home. What was the total distance she traveled?

A) 18 miles

B) 32 miles

C) 48 miles

D) 56 miles

20. An ice chest contains 24 sodas, some regular and some diet. The ratio of diet soda to regular soda is 1:3. How many regular sodas are in the ice chest?

A) 1

B) 4

C) 18

D) 24

CONTINUE

21. What is the area of the shape below?

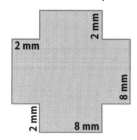

A) 6 mm²

B) 16 mm²

C) 64 mm²

D) 128 mm²

22. Out of 1560 students at Ward Middle School, 15% want to take French. Which expression represents how many students want to take French?

A) $x = 1560 \div 15$

B) $x = 15 \div 1560$

C) $x = 1560 \times 0.15$

D) $x = 1560 \div 100$

23. Solve for x: $5x - 4 = 3(8 + 3x)$

A) -7

B) $-\frac{3}{4}$

C) $\frac{3}{4}$

D) 7

24. The pie graph below shows how a state's government plans to spend its annual budget of $3 billion.

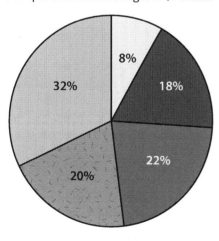

○ Employees ● Education

● Healthcare ○ Pension

● Infrastructure

How much more money does the state plan to spend on infrastructure than education?

A) $60,000,000

B) $120,000,000

C) $300,000,000

D) $600,000,000

25. If a car uses 8 gallons of gas to travel 650 miles, how many miles can it travel using 12 gallons of gas?

A) 870 miles

B) 895 miles

C) 915 miles

D) 975 miles

26. The perimeter of a rectangle is 42 mm. If the length of the rectangle is 13 mm, what is its width?

A) 8 mm

B) 13 mm

C) 20 mm

D) 29 mm

27. A bike store is having a 30%-off sale, and one of the bikes is on sale for $385. What was the original price of this bike?

A) $253.00

B) $450.00

C) $500.50

D) $550.00

28. Justin has a summer lawn care business and earns $40 for each lawn he mows. He also pays $35 per week in business expenses. Which of the following expressions represents Justin's profit after x weeks if he mows m number of lawns?

A) $40m - 35x$

B) $40m + 35x$

C) $35x(40 + m)$

D) $35(40m + x)$

29. Five numbers have an average of 16. If the first 4 numbers have a sum of 68, what is the fifth number?

A) 12

B) 16

C) 52

D) 80

30. Adam is painting the outside walls of a 4-walled shed. The shed is 5 feet wide, 4 feet deep, and 7 feet high. How many square feet of paint will Adam need?

    A) 46 square feet

    B) 63 square feet

    C) 126 square feet

    D) 140 square feet

31. The circle below shows a walking path through a park.

    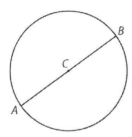

    If the distance from A to B is 4 km, how far will someone travel when they walk along arc AB?

    A) 4 km

    B) 2π km

    C) 8 km

    D) 4π km

32. Alice ran $3\frac{1}{2}$ miles on Monday, and she increased her distance by $\frac{1}{4}$ mile each day. What was her total distance from Monday to Friday?

    A) $17\frac{1}{2}$ mi

    B) $18\frac{1}{2}$ mi

    C) 19 mi

    D) 20 mi

33. A computer store sells both laptops and desktops. On Sunday, the store sold three times as many laptops as desktops. If the store sold a total of 56 computers, how many more laptops did it sell than desktops?

    A) 14

    B) 28

    C) 37

    D) 42

34. A fruit stand sells apples, bananas, and oranges at a ratio of 3:2:1. If the fruit stand sells 20 bananas, how many total pieces of fruit does the fruit stand sell?

    A) 10

    B) 30

    C) 40

    D) 60

35. Which of the following is the y-intercept of the given equation?

    $7y - 42x + 7 = 0$

    A) $(-1, 0)$

    B) $(0, -1)$

    C) $(0, \frac{1}{6})$

    D) $(6, 0)$

36. A 10 L container will hold how much more liquid than a 2-gallon container? (1 gal $= 3.785$ L)

    A) 2.00 L

    B) 2.43 L

    C) 6.22 L

    D) 8.00 L

37. A cyclist is moving down the sidewalk at 15 feet per second. What is his approximate speed in miles per hour?

    A) 10.2 mph

    B) 15.9 mph

    C) 17.1 mph

    D) 22 mph

38. What number is in the hundredths place when 21.563 is divided by 8?

    A) 5

    B) 6

    C) 8

    D) 9

39. If the circumference of a circle is 18π, what is the area of the circle?

    A) 9π

    B) 18π

    C) 27π

    D) 81π

40. In a recent election, 80% of eligible voters cast votes. Hank earns 4,000 votes, which is 40% of the vote. How many eligible voters live in the city?

    A) 5,000

    B) 8,000

    C) 10,000

    D) 12,500

41. How many $\frac{1}{3}$-cup servings can be poured from $5\frac{2}{3}$ cups of juice?

    A) $1\frac{1}{9}$

    B) 5

    C) $15\frac{1}{3}$

    D) 17

42. Simplify: $\frac{7}{8} - \frac{1}{10} - \frac{2}{3}$

    A. $\frac{1}{30}$

    B. $\frac{13}{120}$

    C. $\frac{4}{21}$

    D. $\frac{4}{105}$

Science

Directions: Read the question carefully, and choose the best answer.

1. Which of the following chambers of the heart pumps oxygenated blood to the rest of the body?

    A) left atrium

    B) right atrium

    C) left ventricle

    D) right ventricle

2. An organism has eight pairs of chromosomes. How many chromosomes does each egg or sperm cell contain?

    A) 4

    B) 8

    C) 16

    D) 32

3. After air is inhaled through the mouth, nose, and throat, which of the following structures does it travel through?

    A) alveoli

    B) bronchi

    C) bronchioles

    D) trachea

4. The identity of an element is determined by its number of

    A) neutrons.

    B) nuclei.

    C) protons.

    D) electrons.

5. Which of the following cells carry oxygen?

    A) leukocytes

    B) thrombocytes

    C) erythrocytes

    D) plasma cells

6. Oxygen is exchanged between blood and tissues at which of the following areas?

    A) capillaries

    B) veins

    C) ventricles

    D) arteries

7. How many electrons are included in the double bond between the two oxygen atoms in O_2?

    A) 2

    B) 4

    C) 6

    D) 8

8. Which of the following is the anterior bone of the lower leg?

    A) ulna

    B) fibula

    C) tibia

    D) radius

9. Which of the following regions of the brain is the active link between the endocrine and nervous systems?

    A) cerebellum

    B) pons

    C) cerebrum

    D) hypothalamus

10. How many electrons are needed to complete the valence shell of the halogens?

    A) 1

    B) 2

    C) 6

    D) 7

11. The codon for the amino acid methionine is AUG. Which anticodon would be found on the tRNA that carries methionine?

    A) AUG

    B) TAC

    C) UAC

    D) TUG

12. Which of the following joints is formed by the humerus and the ulna?

    A) ball-and-socket joint

    B) hinge joint

    C) saddle joint

    D) gliding joint

13. Which of the following is the process that produces a liquid from a gas?

    A) vaporization

    B) condensation

    C) sublimation

    D) melting

14. In which region of the small intestine are most of the nutrients absorbed?

    A) jejunum

    B) ileum

    C) duodenum

    D) colon

15. What state of matter has a definite shape and definite volume?

    A) solid

    B) liquid

    C) gas

    D) plasma

16. Which of the following macromolecules is broken down by trypsin?

    A) protein

    B) lipid

    C) nucleic acids

    D) carbohydrates

17. Which of the following supplies blood to the lower body?

    A) superior vena cava

    B) inferior vena cava

    C) iliac artery

    D) aortic arch

18. Which type of cell is responsible for the degradation of bone tissue?

    A) osteoclasts

    B) osteoblasts

    C) osteocytes

    D) lining cells

19. The elements in Group 1 have _____ valence electrons and are _____ reactive than the elements in Group 2.

    A) zero; more

    B) zero; less

    C) one; less

    D) one; more

20. Which of the following is NOT an example of the end result of a negative feedback loop?

    A) release of oxytocin during childbirth

    B) vasoconstriction during an incident of low blood pressure

    C) stimulus of sweat glands in thermoregulation

    D) insulin production and storage of glucose during digestion

21. Consider a prokaryotic organism that typically lives in a 10 percent saline concentration environment. Which of the following environments would cause the organism to lose mass at the greatest rate due to osmosis?

    A) a solution of pure water

    B) a solution of 3 percent saline concentration

    C) a solution of 10 percent saline concentration

    D) a solution of 20 percent saline concentration

22. Which of the following is NOT present in an animal cell?

    A) nucleus

    B) mitochondria

    C) cytoplasm

    D) cell wall

23. Which of the following elements is the most electronegative?

A) chlorine

B) iron

C) magnesium

D) silicon

24. Which of the following choices would contain the code for making a protein?

A) mRNA

B) tRNA

C) rRNA

D) DNA polymerase

25. The graph below shows the solubility of several salts at a range of temperatures.

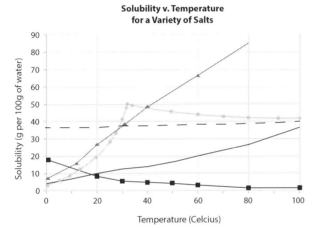

Solubility v. Temperature for a Variety of Salts

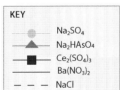

Which of the salts on the graph has the greatest solubility at 50°C?

A) Na_2SO_4

B) NaCl

C) $Ba(NO_3)_2$

D) Na_2HAsO_4

26. The mitral valve transports blood between which of the following two regions of the heart?

A) aorta and left atrium

B) aorta and right atrium

C) right atrium and right ventricle

D) left atrium and left ventricle

27. Which of the following statements best defines a scientific model?

A) a real-world example of a theory

B) a simplification or metaphor for an observed phenomenon

C) a proposed explanation for an observed phenomenon

D) a statement about a fundamental aspect of the universe

28. A chemistry student is conducting an experiment in which she tests the relationship between reactant concentration and heat produced by a reaction. In her experiment, she alters the reactant concentration and measures heat produced. Which of the following is the independent variable in this experiment?

A) reactant concentration

B) reaction rate

C) amount of heat produced by the reaction

D) product concentration

29. Which of the following is NOT a homogenous mixture?

A) air

B) sandy water

C) brass

D) salt dissolved in water

30. Alleles for brown eyes (B) are dominant over alleles for blue eyes (b). If two parents are both heterozygous for this gene, what is the percent chance that their offspring will have brown eyes?

A) 50

B) 66

C) 75

D) 100

CONTINUE

31. How many neutrons are in an atom of the element $^{88}_{38}$Sr?

A) 38

B) 88

C) 50

D) 126

32. The graph shows the temperature of water as heat is added.

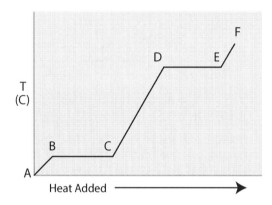

Which of the following processes is occurring between points B and C?

A) boiling

B) melting

C) deposition

D) sublimation

33. Which of the following is a decomposition reaction?

A) $2Na + Cl_2 \rightarrow 2NaCl$

B) $Zn + 2HCl \rightarrow ZnCl_2 + H_2$

C) $CH_4 + 2O_2 \rightarrow CO_2 + 2H_2O$

D) $H_2CO_3 \rightarrow H_2O + CO_2$

34. Which ion has the greatest number of electrons?

A) Ca^{2+}

B) Cl^-

C) Ca^+

D) P^{3-}

35. Damage to the parathyroid would most likely affect which of the following?

A) stress levels

B) bone density

C) secondary sex characteristics

D) circadian rhythms

36. Which of the following is the final vessel through which semen must pass before being expelled from the body?

A) ejaculatory duct

B) penile urethra

C) membranous urethra

D) vas deferens

37. Which of the following groups of bones are part of the axial skeleton?

A) pectoral girdle

B) rib cage

C) arms and hands

D) pelvic girdle

38. Which of the following is NOT a type of white blood cell?

A) helper T-cell

B) plasma cell

C) antibody

D) phagocyte

39. Which of the following is NOT a function of the pituitary gland?

A) receive and interpret internal and external stimuli from sensory nerves

B) release trophic hormones to trigger other glands to produce hormones

C) store hormones from the hypothalamus and release as needed

D) produce hormones and send to target cells via the bloodstream

40. What type of reaction is shown below?

$Zn + CuCl_2 \rightarrow ZnCl_2 + Cu$

A) synthesis reaction

B) decomposition reaction

C) single-displacement reaction

D) double-displacement reaction

41. Which of the following is NOT a hormone-producing gland of the endocrine system?

    A) prostate

    B) pituitary

    C) adrenal

    D) thyroid

42. Mature red blood cells have adapted to not contain a nucleus, which allows them to carry more hemoglobin. What happens to red blood cells as a result of this adaptation?

    A) They cannot undergo mitosis.

    B) They have large energy reserves.

    C) They never die.

    D) They reproduce very quickly.

43. Which of the following is the division of the nervous system primarily responsible for regulating all involuntary and subconscious muscle functions?

    A) somatic nervous system

    B) autonomic nervous system

    C) sympathetic nervous system

    D) peripheral nervous system

44. Read the following passage.

    A scientist discovers a new species of snail that lives in the ocean. He tested the ability of this species to handle heat by measuring its growth rate as he increased the temperature of the water. He also tested two different concentrations of salt to determine which type of marine environment the snail would be best suited for.

    Which of the following is the dependent variable in the experiment described above?

    A) salt concentration

    B) temperature

    C) growth rate

    D) number of snails

45. Which of the following polymers is created by joining amino acids?

    A) DNA

    B) lipid

    C) protein

    D) carbohydrate

46. Which type of bond holds the oxygen and hydrogen atoms in water molecules together?

    A) ionic bond

    B) covalent bond

    C) hydrogen bond

    D) metallic bond

47. In the following acid-base reaction, which species acts as an Arrhenius acid?

    $HCl(aq) + KOH(aq) \rightarrow KCl(aq) + H_2O(l)$

    A) HCl

    B) KOH

    C) KCl

    D) H_2O

48. What substance does a Schwann cell secrete that increases the speed of signals traveling to and from neurons?

    A) myelin

    B) cerebrospinal fluid

    C) corpus callosum

    D) collagen

49. The air in the atmosphere is a solution composed of 78.09% nitrogen (N), 20.95% oxygen (O), 0.93% argon (Ar), and 0.04% carbon dioxide (CO_2) by volume. Which of these gases is the solvent?

    A) nitrogen (N_2)

    B) oxygen (O_2)

    C) argon (Ar)

    D) carbon dioxide (CO_2)

CONTINUE

English and Language Usage

Directions: *Read the question carefully, and choose the best answer.*

1. Which word correctly completes the sentence below?

   She told them to _____ their room before they left for the party.

   A) cleaned

   B) tidy

   C) clears

   D) neat

2. Which word correctly completes the sentence below?

   We left for the party, but my sister had to return home because _____ forgot her purse.

   A) he

   B) they

   C) we

   D) she

3. Which of the following is punctuated correctly?

   A) The dentist told her patient he needed to return later in the week because he had more cavities.

   B) The dentist told her patient he needed to return later in the week: because he had more cavities.

   C) The dentist told her patient he needed to return later in the week; because he had more cavities.

   D) The dentist told her patient he needed to return later in the week—because he had more cavities.

4. Which word is misspelled in the sentence below?

   The invitation presented her with a dilemma: should she go the wedding or go out to diner with her sister?

   A) invitation

   B) dilemma

   C) wedding

   D) diner

5. In which of the following sentences does the verb agree with the subject?

   A) The head zookeeper, who has been with the zoo for over twenty years, have agreed to set up a new enclosure for the elephants.

   B) Of all the elephants owned by the zoo, only some has been approved to move to the new enclosure.

   C) The rest of the elephants has been given to a well-respected rescue organization.

   D) The rescue organization, which takes in animals from zoos across the country, has agreed not to sell the elephants to another zoo.

6. Which of the following is a simple sentence?

   A) He threw the ball across the field to his friend.

   B) He threw the ball to the dog, and the dog ran after it.

   C) He threw the ball across the field because he wanted to see if he could.

   D) He threw the ball across the field; it landed in a ditch.

7. Which word correctly completes the sentence below?

   I had worked a very long shift, _____ I still had to run errands after work.

   A) nor

   B) or

   C) but

   D) so

8. Which of the following has the same meaning as the underlined word in the sentence below?

   The customer was <u>irate</u> and shouted angrily at the staff before leaving.

   A) confused

   B) calculating

   C) furious

   D) frightened

9. Which punctuation mark is used incorrectly in the sentence below?

> We agreed that Chris would plan our mom's birthday party, he had already selected a restaurant, and I didn't have time to pick up a gift.

A) the apostrophe in the word *mom's*

B) the comma after the word *party*

C) the comma after the word *restaurant*

D) the apostrophe in the word *didn't*

10. What part of speech is the word *quickly* in the sentence below?

> He ran quickly while training hard for the race that weekend.

A) verb

B) adjective

C) noun

D) adverb

11. Which sentence is irrelevant as part of a paragraph composed of these sentences?

A) My mom took me to see *The Lion King* on Broadway when I was six, and I knew that I belonged on the stage.

B) I used to perform for my parents in our living room, and I knew all the lines to "Circle of Life" by heart.

C) *The Lion King* is the third-longest-running show on Broadway and the highest-grossing musical of all time.

D) Other people may spend a lifetime looking for the right career, but I've wanted to be an actor since I was a little kid.

12. Which of the following is the complete subject of the sentence below?

> The shiny new fire truck visited the local elementary school.

A) fire truck

B) the shiny new fire truck

C) elementary school

D) the local elementary school

13. Which option puts the following sentences in the proper order for clarity and readability?

> My alarm clock didn't go off.
>
> Fortunately, my boss was also running late.
>
> I arrived at work late.
>
> I didn't get in trouble.

A) I arrived at work late because my alarm clock didn't go off. Fortunately, my boss was also running late, so I didn't get in trouble.

B) My alarm clock didn't go off, but I didn't get in trouble because fortunately, my boss was also running late even though I arrived at work late.

C) I didn't get in trouble because I arrived at work late. My alarm clock didn't go off, and fortunately, my boss was also running late.

D) I arrived at work late. Fortunately, my boss was also running late. My alarm clock didn't go off, but I didn't get in trouble.

14. Which of the following is a compound sentence?

A) I forgot my homework because I was in such a hurry to get to the bus stop.

B) I forgot my homework, but my teacher said I can turn it in tomorrow.

C) I forgot my homework on the dining room table next to my backpack and my lunch.

D) I forgot my homework, but I can turn it in tomorrow if I ask my teacher for permission.

15. Which of the following sentences is written in the third person?

A) You need to check on the patient in room 302.

B) Check on the patient in room 302.

C) He checked on the patient in room 302.

D) I will check on the patient in room 302.

16. Which word BEST captures the meaning of *perfunctory* as used in the sentence below?

> The boss's perfunctory apology left her employees feeling that she wasn't taking their complaints seriously.

A) timid

B) complicated

C) bitter

D) disinterested

17. Which of the following sentences is punctuated correctly?

    A) You need to call the lab, check the test results, and contact the patient's doctors.

    B) You need to call the lab check the test results, and contact the patients doctors.

    C) You need to: call the lab, check the test results, and contact the patient's doctors.

    D) You need to—call the lab, check the test results and contact the patients doctors.

18. Which sentence makes the BEST topic sentence?

    A) Giant pandas live solitary lives and roam large tracks of land looking for food.

    B) Many zoos are working to provide natural, more authentic housing for animals.

    C) Natural borders, such as moats and rock walls, can help make animals feel at home.

    D) Sadly, it seems many zoos do not have the funding to build these large habitats.

19. Which of the following correctly completes the sentence below?

    The letters were quite _____ and contained intimate details.

    A) personal

    B) personnal

    C) personnel

    D) personel

20. Which of the following would create a simple sentence if inserted in the blank below?

    He waited _____

    A) for the bus.

    B) for the bus, but it was running late.

    C) for the bus, so he could get to work on time.

    D) for the bus because he had an appointment.

21. Which word correctly completes the sentence below?

    The heart rate _____ for a number of reasons.

    A) veries

    B) varies

    C) varries

    D) varys

22. Which word or phrase from the sentence below is slang?

    He was hyped for the concert and planned to show up early so he wouldn't miss any songs.

    A) hyped

    B) show up

    C) wouldn't

    D) miss

23. Which word BEST captures the meaning of *stringent* as used in the sentence?

    The stringent entrance requirements made it difficult for even the best students to be accepted to the school.

    A) demanding

    B) confusing

    C) despised

    D) forgettable

24. Which choice CORRECTLY follows the rules of capitalization?

    A) Mr. Jones, who is a Senator

    B) the representative from maine

    C) President Clinton

    D) Vice president Biden

25. Which example is a complete sentence?

    A) The girl who always looks out the window during class.

    B) Because he is running late.

    C) Go look for it now.

    D) Under the stars.

26. Which word is an exception to a common spelling rule?

    A) scarves

    B) noticeable

    C) parties

    D) unfortunate

27. Which punctuation mark BEST completes the sentence below?

> I'm not sure how my book ended up at her house but I want it back.

- **A)** .
- **B)** ,
- **C)** ;
- **D)** :

28. What part of speech is the word *expensive* in the sentence below?

> The dress was beautiful, but it was too expensive for her budget.

- **A)** adjective
- **B)** preposition
- **C)** conjunction
- **D)** noun

29. Which of the following is the meaning of the underlined word in the sentence below?

> Cassandra worked very hard to <u>hone</u> her skills as a nurse.

- **A)** build
- **B)** sharpen
- **C)** steady
- **D)** improve

30. Which of the following contains an error in sentence structure?

- **A)** I asked the teacher when the project was due; she said we had two weeks to finish it.
- **B)** I love running, to swim, and also going hiking, but I hate camping.
- **C)** Most of my friends enjoy soccer, but I prefer basketball.
- **D)** The municipal government stated that there would be no budget increase this year.

31. Dr. Jones had a _____ to speak loudly, which often upset people.

- **A)** tendancy
- **B)** tendency
- **C)** tendencie
- **D)** tendincy

32. Which pronoun correctly completes the sentence below?

> _____ believes that going to a party the night before your certification exam is a bad idea.

- **A)** Everybody
- **B)** Something
- **C)** Several
- **D)** Few

33. Which sentence contains an error?

- **A)** Please sit the plate down on the table.
- **B)** She lay the towel on the sand at the beach.
- **C)** Students should raise their hands if they have a question.
- **D)** On Sundays, I lie on the couch and watch TV if I'm not busy.

34. Which of the following is the meaning of the underlined word in the sentence below?

> Omari felt <u>apathetic</u> in his employment, so he decided to quit his job and go to nursing school.

- **A)** motivated
- **B)** dissatisfied
- **C)** indifferent
- **D)** unsure

35. Which word is used incorrectly in the following sentence?

> The members of the orchestra played good last night, so they received a standing ovation.

- **A)** played
- **B)** good
- **C)** received
- **D)** ovation

36. Which words from the following sentence are pronouns?

> I offered to help her study for the test, but she was too busy.

- **A)** I, her, she
- **B)** offered, help, study
- **C)** to, for, but, was
- **D)** test, too, busy

37. Which of the following sentences is grammatically correct?

A) There are too many stares; I'd rather take the elevator.

B) There are too many steers; I'd rather take the elevator.

C) There are too many stairs; I'd rather take the elevator.

D) There are too many stars; I'd rather take the elevator.

38. Select the BEST words for the blanks in the following sentence.

Mateo was _____ busy studying for an exam _____ attend the party with his roommate.

A) too, too

B) two, too

C) to, two

D) too, to

Reading

1. **C)** The first sentence of the passage explains that jazz "reached into many aspects of American culture." The rest of the passage supports this idea by discussing the role of jazz in the growth of urban centers, in the movement for women's rights, and in the Harlem Renaissance.

2. **D)** This sentence is a supporting idea because it provides another reason why jazz is considered influential in American culture.

3. **B)** Expository writing is used to describe, explain, or provide information. It includes a logical sequence of steps or order of events.

4. **A)** The second paragraph describes how jazz music influenced the struggles of two minority groups—women and African Americans.

5. **C)** The organization of the passage is chronological: it traces the popularity of popcorn from the ancient world through the twentieth century and to the modern day.

6. **A)** The last sentence of the third paragraph states that "popcorn continued to rule the snack food kingdom until the rise in popularity of home televisions during the 1950s," suggesting that as people watched more television, they went to the movie less, and thus ate less popcorn.

7. **C)** The passage explains that popcorn is a food that many cultures have eaten and also describes the growth of the popcorn industry over time.

8. **B)** The popcorn industry will likely continue to thrive because every time it has faced a decline, it has come up with a new way to market its product and make it available to consumers.

9. **A)** This passage most likely comes from a short-story collection because it tells the story of an individual. It does not focus on information, processes, or historical events.

10. **D)** The passage describes how Mason makes friends on a bus and on a team. It also states that "people sought out Mason," meaning that people wanted to be around him.

11. **C)** The subject line of the memo is "Personal Use of Computers," and this memo is being sent to department leaders.

12. **D)** The memo states that management will take disciplinary action against employees who use computers for personal matters during work hours. The memo stresses the seriousness of the issue by stating, "These rules must be respected."

13. **C)** This is an example of persuasive writing. The author is arguing for a particular interpretation of historical events. The statement "but people who try to sell you this narrative are wrong" clearly attempts to sway the reader.

14. **A)** The author states, "The Civil War was not a battle of cultural identities—it was a battle about slavery" in an attempt to persuade the reader. The rest of the passage supports this idea.

15. **B)** The author states in the passage that the Civil War was not "a battle of cultural identities [but] ... a battle about slavery." *Slavery* and *slave labor* can be considered synonymous terms.

16. **B)** The passage states that "surgery patients must check in at the Hospital Admissions Desk" before going to the third floor for surgery.

17. **C)** The passage states that the nurse at the Surgery Admissions Desk will "ensure that all required paperwork has been completed before the patient is taken to the Surgery Holding Room."

18. **A)** A primary source is produced by someone with firsthand knowledge of the events being described. Of the choices, only the letter writer was a witness to the Battle of Gettysburg.

19. **C)** Beech trees are included in the list of species found in a temperate deciduous forest.

20. **C)** The transition word *overall* is used to indicate a conclusion or summary.

21. **D)** The entry for short-term memory shows that it begins on page 340.

22. **A)** The temperature −40°F is equivalent to −40°C.

23. **A)** The thermometer currently reads 20°C. If the temperature dropped 10°C, the thermometer would read 10°C, or approximately 50°F.

24. **A)** The diner has the fewest number of bacon slices (nineteen), and bacon slices occupy the smallest slice of the pie chart.

25. **A)** Adding 120 buns to the existing eighty buns would provide enough buns for 200 hamburgers.

26. **A)** There are enough bacon slices to make nineteen burgers, and enough cheese slices to make eighteen burgers (37 ÷ 2 = 18.5). The most hamburgers that Gigi's could make is eighteen.

27. **D)** The context clues *wit* and *flair* suggest the president used engaging wordplay, meaning he was well-spoken.

28. **B)** The passage is primarily informative. However, the author uses humorous language like "floppy satellite dishes" and "the deafening reverberations of the top forty" to entertain readers.

29. **A)** The author is referring to the fact that our ears have another purpose in addition to hearing.

30. **C)** In the second paragraph, the author writes, "You have five balance receptors. Two receptors detect linear motion.... The other three receptors ... work together to detect head rotation."

31. **D)** The first paragraph begins with "Most people think ...." The author goes on to describe external respiration and then asks, "Did you know there are actually two types of respiration in humans?" Finally, the author describes the other type: internal respiration. The author is probably correct in assuming that most people—excluding biologists and medical professionals—have never heard of internal respiration.

32. **A)** The primary purpose of the essay is to inform; its focus is on the two types of respiration. It is not persuasive or advisory. The author is not trying to prove a point.

33. **D)** This is the site of a government agency. This site will focus on studies and factual data rather than personal opinions or consumer products.

34. **C)** All of these titles are subheadings (marked with the letter A or B) that fall under a major heading (marked with a number).

35. **B)** In this passage, bold print is used to make certain words stand out from the rest of the text.

36. **B)** Work through each step.
    1. $20
    2. 20 – 5 = $15
    3. 15 + 20 = $35
    4. 35 – 10 = $25
    5. 25 + 10 = $35
    6. 35 – 30 = **$5**

37. **C)** Work through each step.

1. 3 gallons
2. 3 − 0.5 = 2.5 gallons
3. 2.5 − 1 = 1.5 gallons
4. 1.5 − 0.5 = 1 gallon

38. **A)** The context clue "poor night's sleep" suggests that Elaine was feeling tired.

39. **C)** "Recipes for Common Dishes" is the only heading that is not about an art form.

40. **B)** Work through each step.

1. 0 miles north, 0 miles west
2. 10 miles north, 0 miles west
3. 10 miles north, 5 miles west
4. 8 miles north, 5 miles west
5. 8 miles north, 6 miles west

41. **A)** A deep cut is the only type of injury that would require stitches and not another form of treatment.

42. **D)** The best heading is "Road Trips" because it is the only option that suggests another method of travel.

43. **B)** Work through each step.

1. one red, two green
2. zero red, two green
3. zero red, three green
4. one red, three green
5. one red, four green
6. zero red, four green
7. zero red, three green
8. three red, three green
9. three red, five green

44. **D)** Based on context clues in the passage, it appears that the couple has no schedule, strategy, or set ideas about their travels. Therefore, the word *plan* is used with irony or sarcasm.

45. **C)** The phrase showed up is idiomatic and less formal than the word arrived.

Mathematics

1. **D)** Write a proportion and then solve for *x*:

$$\frac{40}{45} = \frac{265}{x}$$

$$40x = 11{,}925$$

$$x = 298.125 \approx \mathbf{298}$$

2. **C)** Use the formula for percentages:

$$\text{percent} = \frac{\text{part}}{\text{whole}}$$

$$= \frac{42}{48}$$

$$= 0.875 = \mathbf{87.5\%}$$

3. **C)** The digit in the hundredths place is 3.

1230.9<u>3</u>2567

The digit to the right of the hundredths place is 2, which is less than 5. Therefore, the 3 remains the same. The number rounds to **1230.93**.

4. **C)** Use the area to find the length of a side of the square:

$$A = s^2$$

$$5625 \text{ ft}^2 = s^2$$

$$s = \sqrt{5625 \text{ ft}^2} = 75 \text{ ft}$$

Now multiply the side length by 4 to find the perimeter.

$$P = 4s$$

$$P = 4(75 \text{ ft}) = \mathbf{300 \text{ ft}}$$

5. **C)** Use the equation for percentages.

$$\text{whole} = \frac{\text{part}}{\text{percent}} = \frac{45}{0.25} = \mathbf{\$180}$$

6. **B)** Use the equation for percentages.

$$\text{part} = \text{whole} \times \text{percent} = 2000 \times 0.05 = \mathbf{100}$$

7. **A)** The amount of money in Jane's bank account can be represented by the expression 275 + 15*h* ($275 plus $15 for every hour she works). Therefore, the equation 400 = 275+15*h* describes how many hours she needs to babysit to have $400.

8. **B)** Circumference of a circle: $C = 2\pi r$.

$$d = 2r, \text{ so } C = \pi d.$$

$$50 \text{ ft} = \pi d$$

$$d = \frac{50}{\pi}$$

9. **C)** There are twice as many red marbles as blue marbles, so (red) = 2(blue).

The number of blue marbles is 88% the number of green marbles, so (blue) = 0.88g.

Substitute this expression for blue marbles in the one above:

(red) = 2(0.88g)

(red) = 1.76g

The total number of marbles is equal to red plus blue plus green:

(red) + (blue) + g

1.76g + 0.88g + g = **3.64g**

10. **D)** Write each value in decimal form and compare.

$-0.95 < 0 < 0.4 < 0.35 < 0.75$ FALSE

$-1 < -0.1 < -0.11 < 0.8\underline{3} < 0.75$ FALSE

$-0.75 < -0.2 < 0 < 0.6\underline{6} < 0.55$ FALSE

$-1.1 < -0.8 < -0.13 < 0.7 < 0.8\underline{1}$ TRUE

11. **C)**

$\frac{2x + 7}{9} < 2$

Multiply both sides by 9:

$2x + 7 < 18$

Subtract 7 from both sides:

$2x < 18 - 7$

$2x < 11$

Divide both sides by 2:

$x < \frac{11}{2}$

12. **C)** Line segment *MN* begins at 35 mm and ends at 70 mm, so 70 − 35 = 35 mm.

The length of line segment *KL* is 15 mm.

Find the difference.

35 mm − 15 mm = **20 mm**

13. **B)** Multiply the number of bottles by the amount each holds.

$24 \times 0.75 =$ **18**

14. **C)** Subtract 2 from both sides:

$3x + 2 > 5$

$3x > 3$

Divide both sides by 3:

$x > 1$

15. **A)** Add the number of cupcakes he will give to his friend and to his coworkers, then subtract that value from 48.

$\frac{1}{2} \times 48 = 24$

number of cupcakes for his coworkers:

$\frac{1}{3} \times 48 = 16$

$48 - (24 + 16) =$ **8**

16. **A)** In 2003, the profit was about $4 million. In 2004, the profit jumps to just over $6.2 million.

6.2 million − 4 million = **$2.2 million**

17. **A)** The question asks for the difference in profit between 2001 and 2000. In 2001, approximately $2 million was earned, and in 2000, approximately $1 million was earned.

2 million − 1 million = **$1 million**

18. **A)** Use the equation for percentages.

part = whole × percentage = $9 \times 0.25 =$ **2.25**

19. **C)** The 3 legs of the trip make a right triangle.

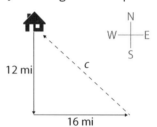

Use the Pythagorean theorem to find the distance she traveled from her final point back to her home:

$a^2 + b^2 = c^2$

$12^2 + 16^2 = c^2$

$144 + 256 = c^2$

$400 = c^2$

$c = 20$

Finally, add the three legs to find the total distance she traveled:

12 + 16 + 20 = **48 miles**

20. **C)** Use a proportion.

$\frac{\text{regular}}{\text{total}} = \frac{3}{4} = \frac{x}{24}$

$4x = 72$

$x =$ **18**

21. **D)** Find the area of the square if it did not have the corners cut out.

$12 \text{ mm} \times 12 \text{ mm} = 144 \text{ mm}^2$

Find the area of the 4 cut-out corners.

$2 \text{ mm} \times 2 \text{ mm} = 4 \text{ mm}^2$

$4(4 \text{ mm}^2) = 16 \text{ mm}^2$

Subtract the area of the cut-out corners from the large square to find the area of the shape:

$144 \text{ mm}^2 - 16 \text{ mm}^2 = \textbf{128 mm}^2$

22. **C)** Use the formula for finding percentages. (Express the percentage as a decimal.)

part = whole × percentage = $\textbf{1560} \times \textbf{0.15}$

23. **A)** Isolate the variable x on one side of the equation:

$5x - 4 = 3(8 + 3x)$

$5x - 4 = 24 + 9x$

$-4 - 24 = 9x - 5x$

$-28 = 4x$

$-\frac{28}{4} = \frac{4x}{4}$

$x = \textbf{-7}$

24. **A)** Find the amount the state will spend on infrastructure and education.

Infrastructure = $0.2(3,000,000,000) = 600,000,000$

Education = $0.18(3,000,000,000) = 540,000,000$

Find the difference.

$600,000,000 - 540,000,000 = \textbf{\$60,000,000}$

25. **D)** Set up a proportion and solve.

$\frac{8}{650} = \frac{12}{x}$

$12(650) = 8x$

$x = \textbf{975 miles}$

26. **A)** Use the equation for the perimeter of a rectangle.

$P = 2l + 2w$

$42 = 2(13) + 2w$

$w = \textbf{8}$

27. **D)** Set up an equation and solve: the original price (p) minus 30% of the original price is $385.

$p - 0.3p = 385$

$p = \frac{385}{0.7} = \textbf{\$550}$

28. **A)** His profit will be his income minus his expenses. He will earn $40 for each lawn, or 40$m$. He pays $35 in expenses each week, or 35w.

profit = $\textbf{40}\boldsymbol{m} - \textbf{35}\boldsymbol{x}$

29. **A)** The average of 5 numbers is the sum of the numbers divided by 5. Multiply the average by 5 to find the sum.

$\frac{\text{sum}}{5} = 16$

sum = $16 \times 5 = 80$

Subtract the sum of the first 4 numbers to find the fifth number.

$80 - 68 = \textbf{12}$

30. **C)** Two of the walls are 5 feet by 7 feet. The other two walls are 4 feet by 7 feet. Therefore, the total area of the four walls is:

$2(5)(7) + 2(4)(7) = 70 + 56 = \textbf{126 ft}^2$

31. **B)** Find the circle's radius.

$4 \text{ km} \div 2 = 2 \text{ km}$

Use the radius to find the circumference of the circle.

$C = 2\pi r = 2\pi(2) = 4\pi$

Arc AB is a semicircle, which means its length is half the circumference of the circle.

$\frac{4\pi}{2} = \textbf{2}\boldsymbol{\pi} \textbf{ km}$

32. **D)** Find the daily distance by adding $\frac{1}{4}$ mile to each day.

Day	Monday	Tuesday	Wednesday	Thursday	Friday
Distance	$3\frac{1}{2}$	$3\frac{1}{2} + \frac{1}{4} = 3\frac{3}{4}$	$3\frac{3}{4} + \frac{1}{4} = 4$	$4 + \frac{1}{4} = 4\frac{1}{4}$	$4\frac{1}{4} + \frac{1}{4} = 4\frac{1}{2}$

Add each daily distance to find the total.

$3\frac{2}{4} + 3\frac{3}{4} + 4 + 4\frac{1}{4} + 4\frac{2}{4} = 18\frac{8}{4} \rightarrow 18 + 2 = \textbf{20}$

33. **B)** Let x = the number of desktops sold.

The store sold three times as many laptops as desktops.

Let $3x$ = number of laptops.

The number of laptops plus the number of desktops is 56.

$x + 3x = 56$

$4x = 56$

$x = 14$

There were 14 desktops sold and $14(3) = 42$ laptops sold.

Subtract to find how many more laptops than desktops sold.

$42 - 14 = \textbf{28}$

34. **D)** Assign variables and write the ratios as fractions. Cross multiply to solve.

Let x = number of apples

$\dfrac{\text{apples}}{\text{bananas}} = \dfrac{3}{2} = \dfrac{x}{20}$

$60 = 2x$

$x = 30$ apples

Let y = number of oranges

$\dfrac{\text{oranges}}{\text{bananas}} = \dfrac{1}{2} = \dfrac{y}{20}$

$2y = 20$

$y = 10$ oranges

Add the number of apples, oranges, and bananas to find the total.

$30 + 20 + 10 = \textbf{60 pieces of fruit}$

35. **B)** Substitute 0 for x and solve for y.

$7y - 42x + 7 = 0$

$7y - 42(0) + 7 = 0$

$y = -1$

The y-intercept is at **(0, −1)**.

36. **B)** Convert gallons to liters.

$2 \text{ gal} \times \dfrac{3.785 \text{ L}}{1 \text{ gal}} = 7.57 \text{ L}$

Subtract to find the difference in liters.

$10 \text{ L} - 7.57 \text{ L} = \textbf{2.43 L}$

37. **A)** Use dimensional analysis to convert feet to miles and seconds to hours.

$\dfrac{15 \text{ ft}}{\text{sec}} \times \dfrac{3600 \text{ sec}}{1 \text{ hr}} \times \dfrac{1 \text{ mi}}{5280 \text{ ft}} \approx \textbf{10.2 mph}$

38. **D)** Divide and find the digit in the hundredths place.

$21.563 \div 8 = 2.6\underline{9}5375$

39. **D)** Use the formula for circumference of the circle to find the radius.

$C = 2\pi r$

$18\pi = 2\pi r$

$r = 9$

Use the radius to find the area.

$A = \pi r^2$

$A = \pi(9)^2$

$A = \textbf{81}\pi$

40. **D)** Hank earned 4,000 votes, which is 40% of the vote.

Write and solve the proportion.

$\dfrac{4{,}000}{x} = \dfrac{40}{100} \rightarrow x = 10{,}000$

10,000 voters is 80% of the total number of eligible voters. Set up another proportion to find the total number of voters.

$\dfrac{10{,}000}{x} = \dfrac{80}{100} \rightarrow x = \textbf{12,500}$

41. **D)** Divide the total amount of juice by the amount in each serving.

$5\tfrac{2}{3} \div \tfrac{1}{3} = \tfrac{17}{3} \div \tfrac{1}{3} = \tfrac{17}{3} \times \tfrac{3}{1} = \textbf{17}$

42. **B)** Convert each fraction to the LCD and subtract the numerators.

$\tfrac{7}{8} - \tfrac{1}{10} - \tfrac{2}{3}$

$= \tfrac{7}{8}\left(\tfrac{15}{15}\right) - \tfrac{1}{10}\left(\tfrac{12}{12}\right) - \tfrac{2}{3}\left(\tfrac{40}{40}\right)$

$= \tfrac{105}{120} - \tfrac{12}{120} - \tfrac{80}{120} = \tfrac{13}{120}$

Science

1. **C)** The left ventricle receives oxygenated blood from the left atrium, then pumps the blood to the rest of the body.

2. **B)** If an organism has eight pairs of chromosomes, it would have a diploid number ($2n$) of 16. The haploid number ($1n$) would be 8.

3. **D)** The trachea, or windpipe, is a passageway for air as it moves from the mouth, nose, and throat to the bronchi.

4. **C)** The number of protons determines which element it is.

5. **C)** Erythrocytes are red blood cells that contain hemoglobin, which is responsible for carrying oxygen within the blood cell.

6. **A)** Capillaries are very small blood vessels found where veins and arteries meet. They are the site of material exchange.

7. **B)** The two oxygen atoms in a covalent double bond share two pairs of electrons, or four total.

8. **C)** The tibia, or shin bone, is the larger of the lower leg bones and is located slightly to the front of the smaller fibula.

9. **D)** The hypothalamus links the nervous and endocrine systems by regulating hormone production of the pituitary gland.

10. **A)** Group 17, called the halogens, have seven electrons in their valence shell and need one electron to complete the shell.

11. **C)** Each tRNA molecule has an anticodon that binds to the complementary codon on the mRNA strand. A bonds with U (not T, as in DNA), U bonds with A, and G bonds with C.

12. **B)** The humerus and ulna connect at the elbow to form a hinge joint.

13. **B)** Condensation is a phase change that occurs when gas, such as water vapor, is converted to liquid, such as water.

14. **A)** The jejunum, the middle section of the small intestine, is the site of most of the food absorption in the body after it is broken down in the duodenum.

15. **A)** A solid has a definite shape and definite volume.

16. **A)** Trypsin is a digestive enzyme that breaks down protein into peptides and amino acids.

17. **C)** The iliac artery receives blood from the aorta to supply blood to the lower body.

18. **A)** Osteoclasts break down and absorb bone tissue.

19. **D)** Group 1 elements contain one valence electron. They are more reactive than Group 2 elements because they have a full valence shell when they lose their one valence electron, meaning they lose that electron very easily.

20. **A)** The release of oxytocin during childbirth is a positive feedback loop because it moves the body further from homeostasis rather than toward it.

21. **D)** Water will leave the cell through osmosis when the concentration of solute outside the cell is greater than that inside the cell. Water will leave the cell when it's placed in a 20 percent solute solution, decreasing the mass of the cell.

22. **D)** The cell wall is the structure that gives plant cells their rigidity.

23. **A)** Electronegativity increases from left to right and bottom to top along the periodic table. Chlorine is higher and more to the right on the table than the other answer choices, so it is the most electronegative.

24. **A)** mRNA is a sequence of nucleotides in which each triplet codes for a particular amino acid. The sequence of triplets in the mRNA would translate into the sequence of amino acids that make up a protein.

25. **D)** The solubility for Na_2HAsO_4 at 50°C is around 55 grams/100 grams of water. This is the highest for the solutes listed on the graph.

26. **D)** These two structures form a junction at the mitral valve.

27. **B)** Scientific models are simplifications or metaphors for observations that allow the observations to be more easily understood.

28. **A)** The independent variable is deliberately changed in the course of the experiment.

29. **B)** Sandy water is not a homogenous mixture. Sand and water can be easily separated, making it a heterogeneous mixture.

30. **C)** The Punnett square shows that there is a 75 percent chance the child will have the dominant B gene and thus have brown eyes.

	B	b
B	BB	Bb
b	Bb	bb

31. **C)** Subtracting the atomic number from the mass number gives the number of protons: A – Z = 88 – 38 = 50.

32. **B)** Solid ice is melting into liquid water between points B and C.

33. **D)** This is a decomposition reaction where one reactant breaks apart into two products.

34. **C)** Ca^+ has nineteen electrons. All the other ions have eighteen electrons.

35. **B)** The parathyroid controls calcium and phosphate levels, which are maintained by producing and reabsorbing bone tissue.

36. **B)** Both urine and semen travel through the penile urethra, the longest portion of the male urethra, to be expelled through the urethral opening.

37. **B)** The rib cage, which consists of the ribs and the sternum, is part of the axial skeleton.

38. **C)** Antibodies are proteins produced by plasma cells.

39. **A)** The pituitary gland does not play a role in processing sensory information.

40. **C)** The zinc and copper reactants switch places with each other on the product side, so this is a single-displacement reaction.

41. **A)** The prostate is an exocrine gland that secretes the alkaline fluid found in semen. It does not produce hormones.

42. **A)** Red blood cells are created in bone marrow instead of through mitosis. They are the only type of cell to be created in this way. Without a nucleus, red blood cells are unable to undergo mitosis.

43. **B)** The autonomic nervous system regulates involuntary functions of the heart, digestive tract, and other smooth muscles; it is further subdivided into the sympathetic and parasympathetic nervous systems.

44. **C)** The growth rate is the variable that is dependent on the changes to water temperature and concentration of salt in the water.

45. **C)** Proteins are built by joining amino acids.

46. **B)** The oxygen and hydrogen in a water molecule share electrons, creating a covalent bond.

47. **A)** An Arrhenius acid is a species or substance that produces H^+ ions. Strong acids like hydrochloric acid (HCl) produce hydrogen ions (H^+).

48. **A)** Schwann cells secrete myelin, which forms a sheet around the neuron and allows the electrical signal to travel faster.

49. **A)** Nitrogen (N) is the largest component of the mixture and therefore is considered the solvent.

English and Language Usage

1. **B)** *Tidy* is the only choice that is a verb and is in the infinitive form (*to tidy*).

2. **D)** The female third-person pronoun *she* replaces "my sister."

3. **A)** No punctuation is needed to join a dependent clause ("because he had more cavities") to the end of an independent clause.

4. **D)** *Diner* should be spelled "dinner." A diner is a restaurant; dinner is the meal eaten in the evening.

5. **D)** The singular subject *organization* agrees with the singular verb *has*.

6. **A)** A simple sentence has one independent clause and no dependent clauses.

7. **C)** *But* links two ideas that contrast each other, suggesting that one thing has to be done in spite of the other.

8. **C)** A customer who is "shouting angrily" is furious.

9. **B)** The comma after *party* creates a comma splice, where two independent clauses ("We agreed that Chris would plan our mom's birthday party" and "he had already selected a restaurant") are joined with a comma but no conjunction.

10. **D)** The word *quickly* is an adverb that describes the verb *ran*.

11. **C)** The paragraph is about a child's wish to be an actor. All the sentences relate to this topic except choice C, which does not mention the child.

12. **B)** The complete subject is the simple subject (*fire truck*) and all of its modifiers (*the, shiny, new*).

13. **A)** Choice A combines the sentences in a way that accurately describes the logical relationship between events and also uses clear, grammatically correct sentences and proper punctuation.

14. **B)** A compound sentence has two independent clauses ("I forgot my homework") and ("my teacher said I can turn it in tomorrow") connected by a comma and a coordinating conjunction (but).

15. **C)** *He* is a third-person pronoun, *you* is a second-person pronoun, and *I* is a first-person pronoun. In choice B, the subject *you* is implied.

16. **D)** The context clue "she wasn't taking their complaints seriously" suggests that the boss was disinterested, or not interested, in making a real apology to her employees.

17. **A)** Choice A includes commas to set apart the items in a list and does not include unnecessary punctuation to introduce the list.

18. **B)** This sentence introduces a topic (housing for animals in zoos) that could be explored in a passage. Choices A and C would work best as supporting details. Choice D belongs at the end of a passage because it contains references to previously discussed details.

19. **A)** *Personal* means "something private"; *personnel* are people employed by an organization.

20. **A)** Adding the phrase "for the bus" creates a simple sentence with only one independent clause and no dependent clauses.

21. **B)** The correct spelling is *varies* (the singular version of the verb "to vary").

22. **A)** *Hyped* is a slang term that means "excited."

23. **A)** If "even the best students" can't gain acceptance to the school, the entrance requirements must be demanding, or difficult to achieve.

24. **C)** *President Clinton* is the choice that is properly capitalized. The name and position are capitalized.

25. **C)** The sentence "Go look for it now" is an independent clause that has a subject (implied *you*) and a verb (*go*). Choice A is a noun phrase, and choice D is a prepositional phrase. Choice B is a dependent clause.

26. **B)** The word *noticeable* is an exception to the rule that the final *e* is dropped before adding a suffix that begins with a vowel (drive + ing = driving; observe + ance = observance).

27. **B)** A comma is used to separate two independent clauses with a conjugation (*but*).

28. **A)** The word *expensive* is an adjective that describes *dress*.

29. **B)** To *hone* is "to sharpen." *Build* and *improve* are close in meaning to *hone* but are not synonyms. *Steady* is unrelated.

30. **B)** This sentence does not use parallel structure. A better version is "I love running, swimming, and hiking, but I hate camping."

31. **B)** Choice B, *tendency*, is correct.

32. **A)** The singular indefinite pronoun *everybody* agrees with the singular verb *believes* and makes sense in this context.

33. **A)** The intransitive verb *sit* is used incorrectly here. The writer should have used the transitive verb *set*, which means "to put" or "to set something" down, like plates on a table.

34. **C)** *Apathetic* means "indifferent." Omari might also be unsatisfied with his work, but *dissatisfied* is not the best answer here. He is the opposite of *motivated*. If he were *unsure* about his work, he might not be so quick to leave it.

35. **B)** Choice B is correct. *Good* is an adjective, but because it is modifying the verb *played*, it should be replaced with the adverb *well*.

36. **A)** Choice A is correct: *I* and *she* are subject pronouns, and *her* is an object pronoun. In choice B, the three words are verbs. Choice C includes an infinitive (*to*), a preposition (*for*), a conjunction (*but*), and a verb of being (*was*).

Choice D includes a noun (*test*), an adverb (*too*), and an adjective (*busy*).

37. **C)** Choice C correctly uses the word *stairs* to refer to the steps leading up to a higher elevation. Choice A incorrectly uses the homophone *stares*, meaning "to look intensely." Choice B incorrectly uses *steers*, meaning "cows." Choice D incorrectly uses *stars*, meaning "celestial objects," which is a nonsensical choice in the context of this sentence.

38. **D)** The correct answer is *too* and *to*. The adverb *too* correctly modifies the adjective *busy*. *To* combined with *attend* forms the infinitive verb *to attend*.

Made in United States
Orlando, FL
13 March 2025

59423373R00144